CREATE
YOUR OWN
Perfumes
USING *Essential* OILS

CREATE
YOUR OWN
Perfumes
USING ESSENTIAL OILS

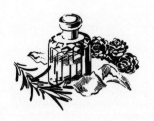

CHRISSIE WILDWOOD

PIATKUS

First published in 1994
by Judy Piatkus (Publishers) Ltd
5 Windmill Street, London W1P 1HF

The moral right of the author has been asserted

A catalogue record for this book is
available from the British Library

ISBN 0-7499-1393-2

Edited by Gillian Haslam
Designed by Zena Flax
Illustrated by Madeleine David

Set in 11½/14pt Garamond by
Action Typesetting Limited, Gloucester
Printed and bound in Great Britain by
Bookcraft Ltd, Midsomer Norton, Avon

Contents

page vii   Acknowledgements

ix   Introduction

xiii   Important Notes

1   *Chapter 1* The Enigmatic Sense

11   *Chapter 2* The Essence of Perfumery

26   *Chapter 3* Aromatic Profiles

55   *Chapter 4* The Alchemist's Workshop

66   *Chapter 5* Creative Blending

84   *Chapter 6* Alluring Skin Perfumes

103   *Chapter 7* Mood-Enhancing Room Scents

127   Bibliography

128   Useful Addresses

129   Index

Acknowledgements

Thank you so much Howard for all the love and home comforts lavished upon me during the birth of this book. Not a word of complaint as I toiled for many hours each day, quite oblivious to everyone else, until it was complete. I also wish to thank Gill Cormode of Piatkus for her scrupulous attention to detail, and my agent Susan Mears for suggesting it in the first place.

He would now study perfumes and the secrets of their manufacture, distilling heavily scented gums from the East. He saw that there was no mood of the mind that had not its counterpart in the sensuous life, and set himself the task to discover their true relation, wondering what there was in frankincense that made one mystical, and in ambergris that stirred one's passions, and violets that woke the memory of dead romance, and in musk that troubled the brain, and champak that strained the imagination; and seeking often to estimate the several influences of sweet-smelling roots, and scented pollen-laden flowers or aromatic balms.

Oscar Wilde
The Picture of Dorian Gray

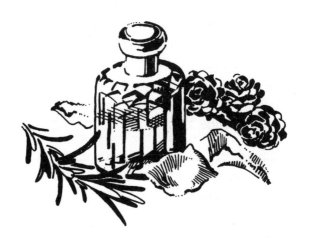

Introduction

Most people would be surprised if they knew exactly what went into some of the big-name perfumes. The beautiful bottles contain exotic cocktails of aroma chemicals, while essential oils distilled from aromatic plants hardly get a look in. To the highly trained nose of the top perfumier, nothing could be more crude than the use of unmodified plant essences.

Unfortunately, most perfumiers are odour-conditioned into believing that synthetic fragrances are superior to those born of a fragrant Earth. In their view, we have become so sophisticated we shy away from those 'raw' scents so beloved by connoisseurs of fragrance in former times, and, they would argue, the fragrance of a synthetic aromatic can be relied upon to smell exactly the same each time it is produced. It is true that the 'bouquet' of an organic essence, just like a good wine, will vary from year to year, depending on the vagaries of the climate and other subtle changes in the environment. To the aromatherapist and the kitchen alchemist, however, such subtle changes simply add to the charm of an essential oil.

If the truth be known, the reason why the modern perfumier is so enamoured of aroma chemicals or 'nature identical' materials (a euphemism for synthetic) is they are less costly to produce than many essential oils. Yet the fragrance of natural rose essence, for example, is so complex that in order for the synthetic counterpart to be convincing, it has to contain a tiny amount of the real thing. In the same way, jasmine cannot be successfully synthesized, at least not to the highly discerning nose, and therefore needs to be heightened with a touch of the natural flower oil. Moreover, as every chemist knows, it is impossible to make a 100 per cent pure chemical. Any synthetic chemical contains a small percentage of undesirable substances not found in the essential oil. In my own experience, synthetic perfume materials are much more likely to cause allergic reactions than essential oils.

Even when natural essences are included in a highly complex formula, the price of the finished product is astronomical compared to the actual cost of the perfume. What you pay for is extravagant packaging, expensive advertising, and a great deal of hype. Perfume manufacturers study the psychology of women, and the increasing number of men, buying perfume. It appears that many people are enchanted by name and price rather than the perfume itself – the more expensive the product, the greater its value in terms of prestige.

As a matter of interest, there are one or two companies marketing perfumes made with the same materials used to create classics such as Chanel No 5, Youth Dew and Opium, but sold at half the price. Even then, they are making a good profit. Most testers would agree that there is very little difference between the real thing and the copy; in fact in some instances, the copy is considered better. So alarmed are the perfume giants by this shattering of illusions, and so powerful are they in the marketplace, that they have successfully banded together to prevent a British discount chainstore from selling big-name perfumes at vastly reduced prices. Yet even though they are aware of the facts, there are still some women who would feel somehow cheated if their lover bought them a smell-alike or a cut-price bottle. It seems that the marketing men will continue to reign supreme over our emotions unless we choose to break free from the chains of manipulation.

I am not suggesting that you should never buy another bottle of perfume again, I am simply asking you to stop for a moment and consider whether you really love the fragrance and feel it is truly worth the money that was spent on it; or in all honesty are you simply spellbound by the power of hard-sell?

It has to be said that organic perfumes are very different from the highly synthetic formulae to which many of us have become accustomed. If you are new to the world of essential oils and aromatherapy, some of the concoctions suggested in this book may take a little getting used to. My aim is to re-educate the average nose in much the same way that the pioneering wholefood enthusiasts succeeded in re-educating many a jaded palate dulled by the blandness of sliced white bread and the overkill of monosodium glutamate.

While there is a plethora of books on both aromatherapy and kitchen cosmetics, the art of perfumery is still a well-kept secret. I hope to encourage you to be wild and creative in the blending of essential oils, which are now widely available from health shops and other outlets. While it cannot be guaranteed that you will compose that masterpiece, once the basic rules are learnt there is plenty of scope for experimenting. You can learn how to make your own personalized fragrances not only to be worn as mood-enhancing skin-perfume (or to scent clothes and hair) but also to vaporize in the home.

Above all, you will discover how to open yourself up to the experience of living fragrance and its power to embrace and heal the emotions. Indeed, there is always an essence, or a blend of essences, to suit your innermost needs — to inspire calmness, exhilaration, sensuality, spirituality and other desirable, yet often elusive, states of mind.

This book is not about traditional aromatherapy. The emphasis is on the psychotherapeutic and sensual aspects of aromatherapy rather than on the treatment of specific physical ailments. If you would like to know more about treating illness with essential oils, there is a suggested list at the end of the book.

I trust that you will enjoy using this book. Do let me know if you create something special — a fragrance in tune with the soul!

Chrissie Wildwood

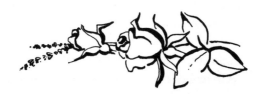

Important Notes

For aromatherapy applications, essential oils are rarely applied neat. They are usually mixed with a good quality base oil such as almond, sunflower or grapeseed in a 1 or 2 per cent concentration, i.e. 1 or 2 drops of essential oil to each teaspoonful (5 ml) of carrier oil. However, the quantity of essential oil in perfume blends is much higher than this, i.e. 10 drops of essential oil to 5 ml of carrier. Therefore, if you have very sensitive skin or know you have an allergy to commercial perfume, you may not be able to wear natural skin-perfumes. You could, however, use room scents instead, or perhaps perfume your clothes (outer garments only) or hair. Indeed, anyone intending to wear perfume long-term would be advised not to apply it to the skin *every* day but to use other methods as well, as overuse of any perfumed product, whether nature of synthetic, can lead to skin sensitivity. If in doubt about using an essential oil (or a blend) for the first time, especially if you have sensitive skin, carry out a patch test.

Patch test

Put a dab of the test oil (or blend) on the inside of your elbow, on the pulse point on your wrist or into the dimple behind your ear. Leave unwashed for 24 hours. If there is no reaction such as itching or redness and if the skin feels comfortable, then go ahead and use that particular oil or blend.

Pregnancy and nursing mothers

It is my own belief that all perfumes, natural or synthetic, should be avoided during pregnancy and whilst breast-feeding. Due to their tiny molecular structure, plant essences and many aroma chemicals can enter the skin and find their way into the bloodstream and body fluids. Many can also cross the placental barrier. Although there is no hard evidence to suggest that mothers and babies have been harmed by perfumes (though there is a murmur in the USA), I still feel it is best to err on the side of caution at this special time, and perhaps to enjoy room scents instead.

Toxic essential oils

It is of great concern that a number of potentially hazardous essential oils are readily available to the public. And worse still, some aromatherapy books advocate the home use of a few of these oils. I trust the following information will serve as a useful source of reference:

Ajowan – possible mucous membrane and skin irritant.

Almond, Bitter – contains prussic acid (cyanide!).

Aniseed – toxic.

Balsam of Peru – potential skin irritant. Use only as a room scent.

Basil, Exotic (*Ocimum basilicum var. basilicum*) – highly toxic to the skin. Use **French Basil** (*Ocimum basilicum var. album*) instead. However, I no longer advocate skin applications of French basil either as in my experience, this too causes skin reactions in a number of people. Use only as a room scent.

Birch, Sweet (*Betula lenta*) – toxic. Not to be confused with **White Birch** (*Betula alba*) which is safe to use.

Boldo Leaf – highly toxic.

Broom, Spanish – highly toxic.

Buchu – suspect until further research is carried out.

Calamus – possible carcinogen.

Camphor, Brown or **Yellow** – carcinogenic. Not to be confused with **White Camphor** (rectified camphor) which is safe in low concentration. All three grades are distilled from crude camphor crystals.

Cassia – powerful skin and mucous membrane irritant.

Chervil – possible carcinogen.

Cinnamon bark – skin and mucous membrane irritant. Use only as a room scent.

Clove – skin irritant and mucous membrane irritant. Use only as a room scent.

Cumin – photo-toxic. The oil may cause dermatitis if applied to the skin shortly before exposure to sunlight.

Deertongue – powerful skin and mucous membrane irritant.

Elecampane (also known as Inula) powerful skin irritant. Use only as a room scent.

Hyssop – may induce epileptic fits in prone subjects.

Jaborandi – highly toxic.

Mugwort – highly toxic.

Narcissus – not recommended for home use as the scent may cause headaches and vomiting.

Oregano – powerful skin and mucous membrane irritant.

Pennyroyal – highly toxic.

Rue – highly toxic.

Sage, Common (*Salvia officinalis*) – toxic. However, **Spanish Sage** (*Salvia lavandulaefolia*) is considered to be safer for home use. Nevertheless, I do not recommend the home use of sage oil at all. Not to be confused with **Clary Sage** (*Clary sclarea*) which is non-toxic.

Santolina – toxic.

Sassafras – carcinogenic.

Savine – highly toxic.

Savory, Summer – powerful skin irritant.

Savory, Winter – powerful skin irritant.

Tansy – toxic.

Tarragon – possible carcinogen.

Thuja – toxic.

Tonka Bean – a dermal toxin. Use only as a room scent.

Wintergreen – toxic. The oil is also an environmental hazard, polluting marine life.

Wormseed – highly toxic.

Wormwood – toxic.

Falsification of melissa oil: True melissa oil is extremely difficult to obtain as so little is produced. When it is available, the oil is very pricy. Most of the so-called melissa oils on the market are blends of infinitely cheaper oils such as lemongrass, lemon and citronella. Rather than be hoodwinked by unscrupulous suppliers, do not use this oil. Only when you have smelled true melissa oil and compared it to the falsified versions will you be able to tell the difference.

Amber: If you come across this oil, be suspicious. It is almost certain to be a synthetic compound or a blend of clary sage and benzoin (a vanilla-like resinoid). As far as I am aware, true amber, from the fossilized resin, is unobtainable. Ambergris (a pathological substance excreted from the whale) is also known as 'amber' and is an extremely costly material used in high class perfumes.

1 The Enigmatic Sense

Fragrance is like music to the sense of smell, evoking emotions, memories and imagery. Yet being the most abstract of the senses, were you to try to describe a particular perfume, you would be lost for the exact word. At best, you might compare it with other scents, or with textures, colours, shapes, sounds or tastes – or even with a certain atmosphere or 'spirit of place'. For instance, a perfume may smell sweetly mellow with a hint of vanilla fudge, or sharp and fruity with a rounded edge, or, more imaginatively, raucous like a scarlet-clad trumpet player, or ethereal like a misty walk in the wildwood. The mute language of fragrance may summon up an elusive déjà vu sensation – 'It reminds me of something, but I can't think what'. Or it may be much more precise, reminding you of first love perhaps, or a childhood visit to a well-loved grandmother who always smelled of Pears soap and fairy cakes.

We need not have smelled a particular fragrance in order for it to work its special magic. Generally speaking, pleasant odours evoke happy memories or feelings, whereas unpleasant ones make us feel uneasy, unless we have learned to associate a particular fragrance with some unpleasant experience. For example, an elderly woman I know cannot abide the scent of rose. One whiff and she is back in the schoolroom, disempowered by the glare of the harsh school-mistress who always smelled of a rose-scented perfume.

Moreover, a certain odour may trigger disharmony for no apparent reason. A friend of mind, for instance, finds the odour of chrysanthemums melancholic. It seems D. H. Lawrence did too, as reflected in the title of his short story *Odour of Chrysanthemums*, a moving tale about a mining disaster. Other sad fragrances, at least to my nose, include the essences of cypress, mimosa and violet leaf.

Intriguingly, many great writers have discovered the power inherent in fragrance to facilitate original thought and creativity. One such notable, the German dramatist and poet Schiller, kept rotten apples in the drawer of his desk and would inhale their pungent aroma whenever he needed to find the right phrase. Proust would travel 100 kilometres to Normandy each spring just to inhale the scent of apple blossom, which he believed gave him direct access to the fount of inspiration. The philosopher Montaigne declared in one of his essays that incense and perfume had the power to comfort, to quicken, to rouse, and to purify our senses so that we might be 'the apter and readier into contemplation'. Moreover, 'Physicians might (in my opinion) draw more use and good from odours than they do. For myself have often perceived, that according unto their strength and qualitie, they change, and alter, and move my spirit and worke strange effects in me.'

And in the not so distant past, George Sand's inspiration was fired by the aroma of tobacco, by the cigars she always smoked whilst writing. And while Kipling's muse resided in rain-damp acacia, 'One whiff is all Arabia', Coleridge's lurked in decay, 'A dunghill at a distance smells like musk, and a dead dog like elder flowers.'

Fantasia

There is no short-term memory with smell. What you encounter may appear to be fleeting, but can be experienced
over and over again. Moreover, within the Eternal Now of
the fathomless psyche there is a place where you may
experience an intermingling of the senses; a pink haze of
fragrance tinkling like wind-chimes, smelling like a cascade of
floating ovals, sweet against the skin, and tasting like sunset.

Those endowed with the condition known as *synesthesia*
will know what I mean. For instance, heavy odours like musk
seed, patchouli and vetiver are commonly perceived as
brownish or olive green, resonating in harmony with the
cello. Lighter fragrances such as bergamot (used to flavour
Earl Grey tea), mandarin and geranium manifest to the syn-
esthete in various hues of bright orange, pink or red, in tune
with the high-pitched sound of the flute or piccolo. Similarly,
composers such as Rimski-Korsakov and Scriabin were
possessed of 'coloured-hearing'. Both associated E major with
bright blue, A-flat major with violet or purple, and D major
with yellow, for example. Although not always in accord,
generally speaking their music-colour sense was in harmony.
In the same vein, some painters are able to 'taste' colour.

It is interesting to note that the hallucinogen LSD triggers
similar, though much more powerful states of synesthesia.
For this reason, the drug was used by the pioneering
symbolist artists whose weird paintings reflect the quest for
'the One hidden in Nature behind the Many'.

Hallucinogenic forays aside for the moment, just how are
odours perceived, and why do they have such a profound
influence upon mood?

Smell and the bodymind

When you hold a fragrant flower to your nose and sniff,
aroma molecules are drawn up in the air stream to a patch

in the roof of the nose. This is the olfactory epithelium, measuring about five square centimetres, which contains up to fifty million odour receptor cells, each bearing microscopic hair-like structures called cilia. These cells (technically speaking they are brain cells) are specialized sensory neurones embedded in a mucous membrane, each connecting directly with the brain by means of a single long nerve fibre. Before the aroma molecules can be detected by the cilia, they must first be dissolved in the mucus. Responses to the aroma molecules are then sent in the form of electro-chemical impulses via the nerve fibres to the olfactory bulb, a part of the brain which actually extends into the nose. The olfactory area of the brain is an aspect of the mysterious limbic system – sometimes called the old brain – which is still largely uncharted territory. It is concerned with our instinctive drives; emotion, intuition, memory, creativity, hunger, thirst, sleep patterns, sex drive, and much more. Through the limbic system, the interconnecting hypothalamus and the pituitary bodies are stimulated, thus causing a cascade of responses in the central nervous system and the entire endocrine (hormonal) system.

From this, we can conclude that any process sending impulses directly to the brain can have far reaching effects upon the body and mind. The healing art of aromatherapy, which combines the use of aromatic plant essences and massage, makes full use of this knowledge.

Pleasing odours – along with other joys such as eating, receiving nurturing massage, falling in love, listening to uplifting music, or being moved by a beautiful landscape – cause the release of certain 'happiness chemicals' such as phenylethylamine (also found in chocolate) and a family of opium-like substances broadly labelled enkephalins and endorphins. Receptors for these brain hormones – including those associated with negative feelings such as fear, anger and depression – are found in other parts of the body, such as the skin, and on cells called monocytes in the immune system. These 'conscious' blood cells circulate freely throughout the body, sending and receiving messages just as diverse as those in the central nervous system. This means that when we are happy, depressed, angry, in love, or whatever, we produce brain chemicals in various parts of the body, meaning that those parts must also be happy, depressed, angry or in love. For this reason, positive emotions strengthen the immune system whereas emotional disharmony weakens our defences. For example, when terminally ill people feel depressed, unloved or fearful, even the pain-killing effect of morphine (derived from opium) is significantly inhibited, as many doctors and nurses working within the hospice movement will verify. However, following successful counselling and a great deal of tender loving care from loved ones and professional carers, sometimes including the use of aromatherapy, the bodymind's own natural opiates are released into the bloodstream, and the need for morphine is often markedly reduced. Moreover, it is also known that the tears of joy and of sorrow are chemically different from each other. Without doubt, the interrelated *bodymind* is a reality.

A palette of odours

Like primary colours, all odours fall into a number of basic categories: floral, minty, camphoraceous, resinous, ethereal (pears), musky, foul, acrid, burnt, mouldy, grassy and so on. In the late 1940s, British chemist J. E. Amoore put forward his *stereochemical* theory of odour, suggesting there may be a connection between the geometric shape of an odoriferous molecule and the odour it produces. Using the 'lock and key' analogy, when an odoriferous molecule comes in contact with a corresponding receptor site on an olfactory neurone, it triggers a nerve impulse to the brain. For example, floral odours are said to have a disc-shaped molecule with a tail, which fits a bowl-and-trough site. Camphoraceous odours have a spherical molecule that fits into an elliptical site, whereas minty odours have a wedge-shaped molecule that fits into a V-shaped site. Some odours appear to fit more than one site at the same time, producing a bouquet effect.

Not all researchers accept the stereochemical theory which is why other more complicated theories abound. It is a fascinating connection, however, for I am one of those synthetists who perceive certain odours in the form of colours and shapes. For instance; the sweet scent of rose essence manifests as a pinky-peach oval; clary sage is bluish-green and shaped like a flying saucer; whereas patchouli smells square with the hue of moist earth. To my nose, pungent odours are dynamic; garlic triggers an array of white stars; the piquant aroma of extra virgin olive oil summons up a short, sharp shock of fizzy bubbles (olive green, of course); whereas the odour of sweaty socks registers as a shoal of sandy-coloured triangles!

Anosmia — the loss of smell

If the olfactory nerve fibres are severed or the nerve pathways damaged, perhaps as a result of head injury, this results in *anosmia*, a major loss of the sense of smell. While it is possible to be born without a sense of smell, anosmia is more often associated with nutritional deficiencies, allergy, nasal polyps (soft fleshy growths, often resulting from a low grade infection), ageing, a brain tumour or exposure to toxic chemicals. Whatever the cause, life without smell can be bleak indeed. Apart from the dangers of being unable to detect the smell of burning, gas leaks or spoiled food, anosmia renders the most ambrosial food tasteless as smell and taste are interrelated functions. About a quarter of sufferers also experience loss of libido.

In her book *A Natural History of the Senses*, American

writer Diane Ackerman cites the case of Judith R. Birnberg who suffered a sudden loss of smell believed to be caused by some unknown allergy. All she can distinguish is the texture and temperature of food. 'I am handicapped... We so take for granted the rich aroma of coffee and the sweet flavour of oranges that when we lose these senses, it is almost as if we have forgotten how to breathe'. Indeed, a woman suffering from anosmia who attended one of my aromatherapy presentations echoed Judith Birnberg's lament, 'Through losing my sense of smell and taste, it seems that life itself now lacks a certain spice and zest.'

Many normal people have 'blind spots' to certain smells of nuances of individual odours, especially to some musks — the sickly sweet and musky aroma of tom cat, for instance. This is known as specific anosmia. In my work as an aromatherapist, I have met two people, both male, who have a specific anosmia to sandalwood essence, even though their sense of smell in other respects is perfectly normal. Yet to the average nose, sandalwood is extremely tenacious. While a few people find it repugnant, detecting a 'sweaty' note, others find the aroma attractive and can testify to its potent aphrodisiac effect.

It is believed that a healthy human nose can detect at least 10,000 different odours. A perfumier may be able to detect several times as many odours as the sense of smell can be enhanced through training. However, when we are subjected to the same smell for even a short time, our sense of smell becomes quickly exhausted as the olfactory cells become 'saturated' and cease to detect it, although we might experience a brief reminder of its presence from time to time. It is also true that if we dislike an odour, it will linger for an eternity!

Another point of interest is that of the many trials carried out at Warwick University by Drs Steve Van Toller and George Dodd, one was of particular note; that we can respond both emotionally and physically to odours so diluted as to be imperceptible to the conscious mind. (Similarly, we can respond to high and low frequency sound — frequencies many animals perceive but which are inaudible to human ears.) Volunteers were connected to an EEG (electroencephalograph) machine which records the electrical activity of the brain as well as subtle skin responses. When exposed to low level fragrance, very clear skin responses were recorded. It appears that the skin acts like antennae, conveying the 'vibes' of the aroma to the central nervous system. Radiological scanning techniques also confirm the brain's registration of odours of which the subject claims not to be aware. From this, we may conclude that even sufferers of anosmia can benefit, albeit on a subliminal level, from the scent of honeysuckle heavy on the air of a summer's evening, or from an aromatherapy treatment or perfume.

Aroma preference and natural body scent

As you may have discovered, the same perfume, aftershave or cologne smells different on different people, especially those of the opposite sex. As the fragrance vaporizes and intermingles with our own body chemistry, different nuances of the scent become apparent. The aroma plays hide-and-seek with the senses — first you smell it, then you don't — until finally it disappears into the ether.

But what is it that determines individual body chemistry? People, as well as animals, secrete subliminally fragrant substances called pheromones — hormone-like substances which influence both sexual attraction and individual body scent. No two people smell exactly alike, though there are similarities between races.

Body scent is also largely determined by the type of food eaten, and influences our aroma preference. People who like spicy food, for example, also plump for strong, penetrating fragrances such as those containing essences of patchouli, sandalwood or ginger. High dairy food consumers prefer light, floral fragrances such as lavender and neroli (orange blossom). The bland but healthy diet of the Japanese, comprised mainly of fish, greens and rice, in conjunction with frequent and meticulous bathing, is one reason why their body odour is virtually non-existent, at least to the noses of many other races. The Japanese are also attracted to delicate fragrances. And while the Eskimo is said to smell 'fishy', the African 'ammoniacal', the rest of the world agrees that the sour 'European' smell is the most offensive.

Emotions, illness, the pill (and other drugs) as well as hormonal changes such as puberty, pregnancy, menstruation and the menopause, all influence body odour and our aroma preference. This explains why the same perfume smells different on each person and why we tend to go off certain perfumes (and also flavours) from time to time and begin to enjoy the ones previously distasteful to us. As we grow older, our bodies secrete different pheromones, and consequently a favourite perfume of our youth may no longer appeal to us in maturity.

It is interesting to note that aroma preference may be vital to the efficacy of an aromatherapy treatment, especially when the sole aim is to heal emotional disharmony. Aroma preference may be less important in the symptomatic treatment of problems such as athlete's foot or scabies though some aromatherapists would disagree. Researchers at Warwick University have recently discovered that if we dislike an aroma, we are able to block its effect on the central nervous system. Yet still there are those who stick rigidly to the idea that rose essence will cure our jealousy, grapefruit our bitterness and jasmine our low self-esteem. The importance of aroma preference and the person's idiosyncratic (therefore unpredictable) response to the aroma is often overlooked. To the intuitive aromatherapist or natural perfumer, aroma preference is an accurate guide to the pattern of the bodymind, for experience has shown that we are instinctively drawn to the fragrance of an essential oil (or blend of oils) that will enhance our physical and emotional well-being.

Odour conditioning or 'fashion' may also play a part in aroma preference which is a pity, because this kind of 'brain washing' inhibits personal expression through the art of creating perfumes from organic essences. True, perfumes made from essential oils do not smell like commercial, highly synthetic formulae. However, as you are about to discover, once drawn into the healing aura of nature's essences born of the synergy of earth, air, sunshine and rain, you will never again become enamoured of the latest highly priced formula, conceived of the synthesis of aroma chemicals, white coats and test tubes.

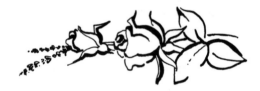

❧ 2 The Essence of Perfumery

A potted history of perfume

To the ancients, the perfume-maker was a weaver of enchantment, a priest or priestess whose alchemical knowledge was employed to create sacred incense with the power to elevate the spirit, linking the human psyche with the power of the gods. As healing and religion were interrelated, the 'smoking' of sick people was used to exorcize evil spirits. In fact, the word 'perfume' is derived from the Latin *per fumum* and means 'through the smoke'.

Throughout the ancient world frankincense resin, extracted from trees grown in south-west Arabia, was traded. It was regarded as the mood-altering substance supreme, the holiest of holy smoke. Frankincense is still burned today in Catholic churches, but I wonder how many priests are aware of its hidden depths? In 1981 scientists in Germany investigated reports that altar boys were getting 'high' on the substance. It was found that when frankincense was burned, it produced trahydrocannabinole, a psycho-active substance known to work strange effects on the imagination.

Perfumes in Ancient Egypt

It was in Ancient Egypt, however, that the use of aromatics reached its zenith. The botanical gardens were a wonder to behold, with many rare and beautiful plants collected from distant lands, such as India and China. It is said that the Egyptian healers were so renowned for their skills that sages and physicians from all over the ancient world came to Egypt to study medicine, perfumery and the Mysteries.

The best known Egyptian incense is Kyphi, a luxurious and heady brew consisting of at least 16 ingredients, including calamus (which contains a narcotic and hallucinogenic substance called asarone), saffron, cassia, spikenard, cinnamon and juniper, all bound together with honey and raisins. Dioscorides, the Greek philosopher writing in the first century AD, called it a perfume welcome to the gods. Kyphi was burnt after sunset, not only to ensure the safe return of the Sun God Ra, but also because its effects were soporific and intoxicating. It was also taken as medicine, or applied externally as a treatment for wounds and skin disorders.

Another mind-bending concoction was Theriaque, said to banish anxiety. It comprised between 57 and 96 ingredients (temple recipes vary), which included myrrh, cinnamon, rush, sweet flag, juniper and cassia and, less aesthetically, serpent skin and spittle!

When Tutankhamen's tomb was excavated in 1922, a little glass pot of unguent was found; although several thousand years old, it was still fragrant with frankincense and spikenard. I once met a forensic scientist fortunate enough to have been present during a research experiment in which a 3,000-year-old mummy was unwrapped. He and his colleagues were intrigued by the aromas of cedarwood and myrrh (the most commonly used aromatics for embalmment) which were still perceptible on the inner bandages.

Until recently, archaeologists believed that the Egyptians

(and other ancient civilizations) used infused oils rather than distilled essences. An infused oil is made by placing plant material in a base of oil or fat and leaving the mixture in the sun for several days, so the base becomes permeated with the aroma. However, according to Dr Jean Valnet, one of the pioneers of modern aromatherapy, the Egyptians used a simple form of distillation to capture essential oils. Water was poured into large clay pots over the plant material (cedarwood for example) and the pot openings were covered in woollen fibres. The pots were heated and the essential oils rose in the steam to become lodged in the wool which was later squeezed to obtain the essential oil.

Similar distillation pots have been found at Tepe Gawra, near ancient Nineveh. They are thought to date back to 3,500 BC, which suggests that the technological achievements of the Mesopotamians have been underrated. However, it was the eleventh century Arab physician Avicenna who perfected the art of distillation to capture the volatile essences of plants. So advanced was his method that the apparatus for distillation has altered very little in 900 years.

Perfumes in Europe

By the twelfth century 'perfumes of Arabia' were famous throughout Europe, for the crusading Knights brought back with them not only exotic and costly perfumes, but also the knowledge of how to distil them.

In sixteenth century Italy, a noble Roman family created a perfume still known by the family name, Frangipani. Made from a cornucopia of ingredients, including almost every known spice, ground iris root and a tinge of civet and musk, the result was an extremely tenacious perfume, similar to the scent of the West Indian flower of the same name.

It was the Italian princess Catherine de Medici in the second half of the sixteenth century who initiated the production of floral fragrances at Grasse in the south of

France where the mild climate and fertile soil helped roses, violets, jasmine and acacia to flourish. In the following century, Grasse became the renowned centre of the perfume industry, an importance it still possesses.

It is a well-documented fact that perfumiers were often immune to the plague, which led to the development of the infamous Four Thieves' Vinegar – a mixture of garlic and aromatic plant essences suspended in vinegar, so-called after a quartet of thieves during the Great Plague in Marseilles in 1722 sprinkled themselves liberally with it before plundering the bodies of the plague victims. All four lived to tell the tale – and to plunder again with impunity!

Despite a strong puritanical influence in Europe which deemed the use of perfume, and indeed all other sensuous pleasures, a source of depravity and shame, the art of perfumery reached its modern climax in nineteenth century Paris. Records show that Napoleon used around sixty bottles of rosemary cologne a month. However, he objected to his beloved Josephine's preference for musk perfume, preferring instead her natural 'three days unwashed' odour: *'Je reviens en trois jours, ne te laves pas!'*. The classic perfume Je Reviens was thus inspired!

In 1868, the British chemist William Henry Perkin succeeded in synthesizing coumarin, a natural perfume chemical, with the scent of newly mown grass. The first perfumes using blends of natural and synthetic odorants were first formulated in the late 1880s by the Frenchman Paul Parquet, who produced classics such as Fougère Royale and Parfum Idéal. By 1921, the incredibly successful Chanel No 5 was born – by mistake! The story goes that Coco Chanel was looking for a fragrance which was evocative of sophisticated freedom. Her perfumiers were experimenting with the new synthetic aldehydes at the time. In one of the test bottles they had prepared for her consideration (the bottle marked No 5), they had accidentally put in about ten times as much aldehyde as intended. However, she adored it, named it after the number on the bottle and started a new trend in synthetic fragrances.

Nevertheless, organic essences still have a role to play in modern perfumery. A few are regarded as precious, for their unique fragrances cannot be successfully reproduced in the laboratory. Rose and jasmine are good examples. But what exactly are essential oils and how are they captured?

The nature of essential oils

Essential oils are the odoriferous liquid components of aromatic plants, trees and grasses. They influence growth and reproduction, attract pollinating insects, repel predators and protect the plant from disease. Unlike 'fixed' or fatty oils, they are highly volatile, which means they evaporate if left in the open air. Many essences have the consistency of water or alcohol — lavender, chamomile and rosemary, for example. Others, such as myrrh and vetiver, are viscous, or thick and sticky, whereas the exquisite rose otto is semi-solid at room temperature but becomes liquid with the slightest warmth.

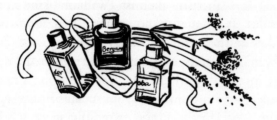

The essences are contained in tiny oil glands or sacs which are concentrated in different parts of the plant. They may be found in the petals (rose), leaves (eucalyptus), roots of grass (vetiver), heart wood (sandalwood), fruit (lemon), seeds (caraway), rhizomes (ginger) or resin (pine) and sometimes in more than one part of the plant. Lavender, for instance yields oil from both the flowers and the leaves, while the orange tree produces three different smelling essences with varying therapeutic properties; the heady bitter-sweet neroli (flowers), the similar though less refined scent of petitgrain (leaves) and the cheery orange (skin of the fruit).

The more oil glands present in the plant, the cheaper the oil, and vice versa. For instance, 100 kilos of lavender yields almost 3 litres of essential oil, whereas 100 kilos of rose petals can yield only half a litre. Essential oils are highly concentrated substances and are therefore rarely used neat, though undiluted lavender essence is sometimes used in aromatherapy as an antiseptic. In perfumery work, plant essences are diluted in oil, wax or alcohol, or partially suspended in distilled water, as explained in chapter 6.

The chemistry of essential oils is complex. They may consist of hundreds of constituents broadly categorized as terpenes, esters, aldehydes, ketones, alcohols, phenols and oxides. This explains why a single essential oil has a wide range of therapeutic properties. Lavender, for example, balances the central nervous system. It is also a wonderful skin healing agent for problems such as athlete's foot, acne and eczema. The essence can also be used in the bath or blended into a massage oil for muscular pain and rheumatism, and much more besides. It is interesting to note that resins such as frankincense and myrrh contain resin alcohols which have a similar chemical structure to human steroids — the male and female hormones. Whether resin alcohols exert a hormone-stimulating effect on humans has not been officially proven, but anecdotal evidence amongst aromatherapists whispers to the affirmative. Of course, much more research into this area is needed before we dare jump to any firm conclusions.

Components of essential oils

The gas chromatograph can separate out the main components of essential oils by looking at the 'chemical fingerprint' produced. However, the pattern of the living essence is complex beyond the chemist's ability to replicate the exact aroma by mixing together the various chemical components. Something is always missing in the 'nature identical' version. However, let's take a look at the main therapeutic effects of the various isolated constituents found in essential oils.

Terpenes: Common terpenes include limonene (an antiviral agent found in 90 per cent of citrus oils), and pinene (an antiseptic found in high concentrations in pine and turpentine oils). Others, such as chamazuline and farnesol (found in chamomile essence), possess remarkable anti-inflammatory and bactericidal properties.

Esters: The most widespread group found in plant essences, which includes linalyl acetate (found in clary sage and lavender), and geranyl acetate (found in sweet marjoram). Esters are fungicidal and sedative, usually with a fruity aroma.

Aldehydes: These substances are found notably in lemon-scented essences such as lemongrass and citronella. Aldehydes generally have a sedative, though uplifting quality.

Ketones: The ketones found in mugwort, pennyroyal, tansy, sage and wormwood are actually toxic, which is why these essences are best avoided by the layperson. However, not all ketones are dangerous. Non-toxic ketones include jasmone found in jasmine, and fenchone in sweet fennel. Ketones ease congestion and aid the flow of mucus, which is why plants and essences containing these substances are helpful for upper respiratory complaints.

Alcohols: Some of the most common terpene alcohols include linalol (found in lavender), citronellol (rose, lemon eucalyptus and geranium) and geraniol (geranium and palmarosa). These substances tend to have good antiseptic and antiviral properties and an uplifting quality.

Phenols: These are bactericidal with a strong, stimulating effect on the central nervous system. However, they can also be skin irritants, especially if isolated from the whole essential oil and used as a single 'active principle'. Common phenols include eugenol (found in clove essence), thymol (found in thyme), and carvacrol (found in oregano). Because phenols are potentially harmful, I have chosen to avoid using essences containing appreciable quantities of these substances, at least for skin use. Clove essence, for instance, can be safely used in room perfumes.

Oxides: These are found in a wide range of essences, especially those of a camphoraceous nature such as rosemary, eucalyptus, tea tree and cajeput. Oxides such as eucalyptol have an expectorant effect.

Essential oils also act on the central nervous system — some will relax (chamomile, lavender, rose otto), others will stimulate (rosemary, black pepper, eucalyptus). A few have the ability to 'normalize'. Hyssop, for example, can raise low blood pressure and lower high blood pressure. Likewise, bergamot and geranium can either sedate or stimulate according to individual needs.

A study in New York's Sloan Kettering Memorial Hospital measured anxiety levels in patients undergoing Magnetic Resonance Imaging, a lengthy and stressful scan used to diagnose life-threatening diseases. When patients sniffed vanilla they experienced 63 per cent less panic than normal. In another study for International Flavours and Fragrances, it was discovered that fragrances containing a tinge of nutmeg helped to reduce stress levels by lowering blood pressure. Similarly, scientists at Yale University found that within a minute of smelling spiced apple, brain waves relaxed and heart rate and blood pressure perceptibly reduced. The aroma also helps stave off panic attacks in susceptible subjects.

As discussed in the previous chapter, the bodymind effect takes place when an essence is inhaled, and an individual responds to its aroma. However, we also know that essential oils have a tiny molecular structure which enables them to pass through the skin's hair follicles which contain sebum, an oily liquid with which they have an affinity. From here they diffuse into the bloodstream or are taken up by the lymph and interstitial fluid (a liquid surrounding all body cells) to other parts of the body from where they act in the manner of a biological catalyst, triggering the body's immune defences. At the same time, when inhaled, the aromatic molecules may also reach the bloodstream via diffusion across the tiny air sacs in the lungs.

Extracting essential oils

The most classic method of extraction is steam distillation. Plant material is piled into a still and subjected to concentrated steam, which acts to release the essential oils from the plant cells. The aromatic vapour travels along a series of glass tubes which form a condenser. The oil is then easily separated from the water by siphoning off through a narrow-necked container. The remaining water may form a beautifully fragrant by-product; rosewater, orange flower water and lavender water are well-known examples.

The essences of citrus fruits such as orange, lemon, bergamot and mandarin are found in the rind, so these can be obtained by a simple process known as expression. Although this was once carried out by hand (by squeezing the rind), machines using centrifugal force are now used instead.

A virtually obsolete method of extraction is called *enfleurage*. Animal fat, usually purified lard, is used to absorb the essences which are then separated from the fat by alcohol. Essences readily dissolve in alcohol, but fat does not. The alcohol is then evaporated off, leaving behind the essential oil. This method is still employed by some perfumiers to capture the fragrances of flowers such as jasmine, orange flower and tuberose, whose fragrances would be spoiled by the intense heat of distillation. If you can actually find such an extraction, it will be labelled *enfleurage absolute*, not 'essential oil', and will cost a fortune. Very few (if any) of these extractions reach the essential oil suppliers. Of course, the use of animal fat will be off-putting to the vegetarian. Although beeswax or vegetable oil could be used instead, I have yet to come across such a product.

The high cost of this labour-intensive and time-consuming method has led to the wide use of solvents such as hexane and petroleum ether as a means of capturing the exquisite essences of certain plants — yet the *enfleurage* process gives a higher yield. Solvent-extracted oils are available from essential oil suppliers and are labelled 'absolute' or, if extracted from gums and resins such as benzoin or Peru balsam, 'resinoid'. The first stage of this process produces a salve-like solid known as a concrete which is treated with alcohol to separate the plant wax from the volatile oil. Though generally more expensive than most essential oils (with the exception of rose otto and neroli), solvent-extracted oils are not as costly as the *enfleurage* absolutes.

However, I avoid the use of absolutes and resinoids in aromatherapy treatments because many of these oils contain traces of solvent and other substances not found in essential oils. Another concern is the fact that potentially harmful solvents may end up in the atmosphere, perhaps as a result of discarding the solvent-soaked plant material onto the rubbish tip (the extraction process itself is carried out in sealed containers, the solvent being continuously recycled).

To my mind, it would not conform to the philosophy of aromatherapy, which professes to be 'holistic' and in harmony with nature, to use anything other than pure essential oils captured by steam distillation or expression rather than potentially toxic solvents. However, for perfumery purposes it is difficult not to concede, for many of the absolutes smell exquisite. Nevertheless, there is a choice of perfumery materials for the blends suggested in Chapters 6 and 7, so you can avoid using solvent-extracted oils if you wish.

The most recent method of obtaining wonderful aromas equivalent to the absolutes is low-temperature liquid carbon dioxide extraction. These substances are entirely free of unwanted solvent residues. Though an expensive process at present, carbon dioxide extraction is generally regarded as a cleaner alternative to the use of chemical solvents. The drawback is that very few suppliers stock these oils.

Home distillation of essential oils

Although I am often asked how to distil essential oils at home, I am far from convinced that this would be a practicable option. For a start, to obtain a 'kitchen table' still would be an amazing accomplishment in itself since they are so hard to come by. Modest sized distillation apparatus can be bought from laboratory equipment suppliers *only* if you have a special commercial licence. Should you succeed against all odds, you may then find yourself the subject of investigation by Customs and Excise — after all, how can you prove you are not also distilling intoxicating liquor?

Be that as it may, some books explain how to rig up a simple still for producing aromatic waters such as lavender water or rosewater. It is possible to produce usable floral waters by the method advocated, but it is an extremely time-consuming process with little return for one's efforts. One source even suggests that you can capture a pure essential oil by the same process. I am deeply sceptical about this; the reasons will become clear once the process has been explained.

Fill a large enamel kettle with your chosen aromatic plant material — lavender, rosemary or rose petals, for example. Pour in as much water as the kettle can hold. Place on the hob and attach a length of plastic tubing (the type used for wine-making) to the spout. Fill a bowl with ice and put this on a low table or short kitchen stool next to the cooker. Place a jug on the floor, near the table or stool. Bend the tubing somewhere in the middle, resting the kink in the ice, then put the end of the tubing into the jug on the floor.

Bring the kettle to the boil, then reduce the heat so the water is kept at a very low simmer for at least an hour (one authority suggests three hours). The steam that travels along the tubing will carry the essential oil droplets. The steam is cooled by the ice, which acts as a condenser, and the result-ing aromatic water drips into the jug.

You can stop at this point and will retrieve the fragrant water, albeit a tiny quantity, and will use it as a skin tonic or as a base for one of the aromatic concoctions suggested in Chapters 6 and 7. If, however, you are a miracle worker, use an eye dropper to remove the essential oil which will float on the top. However, there will be very little essential oil as it takes *at least* six pounds of rose petals (a pro-hibitive quantity for most people) to produce a couple of pints of lightly fragrant water, and very much more than this to produce less than a teaspoonful of rose essence. Moreover, since plant material is so bulky, you would be hard pushed to pack just one pound of it into a kettle — and don't forget, there needs to be some space left for the water.

Rosewood essence

Although rosewood essence is popular with both aromatherapists and perfumiers, much of the oil on the market is captured from trees from the rapidly diminishing rainforests of Brazil. Therefore, if you care about our planet, I hope you will avoid the use of rosewood, sometimes labelled *Bois de Rose.*

Organically produced essences

Not all essential oils are produced by organic methods, i.e. extracted from plants grown without the use of chemical fertilizers and poisonous sprays. Oils labelled 'organic' tend to be of the herb variety, such as lavender, rosemary, marjoram and chamomile, though some oils are distilled from wild plants, extracted from disease-resistant trees such as pine or cypress, or produced in countries where chemical sprays and fertilizers are not in general use.

Unfortunately, not all essential oil suppliers are honest. Some will charge an inflated price for an 'organic' oil – ylang ylang is a good example, where most, if not all, of the ylang ylang oil on the market is organic in the sense outlined above. Or you may be hoodwinked into paying extra for an 'organic' jasmine or rose absolute, when no such oil exists. True, all essential oils are organic in the sense that they are obtained from living plants rather than produced in the laboratory, but the word 'organic' is malleable on the tongue of the dishonest merchant. Moreover, some unscrupulous suppliers may pass off a synthetic or an adulterated essential oil for the real thing. Costly essences such as neroli and rose are sometimes tampered with in this way.

Buying essential oils

In the Useful Addresses section I have listed a few reputable essential oil suppliers, though of course there are many others. The advantages offered by mail order suppliers over retail outlets include a wider range of oils, lower prices on larger quantities and trade discount for aromatherapists. However, if you are unfamiliar with essential oils, it is best to obtain your initial purchases from a health shop or from a well respected herbal supplier. This will give you the opportunity to smell the oils first and buy only those you like.

Diluted oils

Do check that an essential oil labelled as such is in fact 100 per cent essential oil and not one that has been diluted in almond oil (this is sometimes the case with expensive oils such as rose or neroli). Such dilutions are only useful for aromatherapy massage.

Storage and shelf life of essential oils

Storage is very important. Essential oils should be sold in well-stoppered dark glass bottles and stored away from light, heat and damp, which can adversely affect them. Avoid essential oils sold in bottles with a rubber-tipped dropper. Certain essences, cedarwood in particular, can cause rubber to perish into a sticky mess.

In theory, most essential oils will keep for several years, except for the citrus oils, which begin to deteriorate after about six months. Bergamot essence, however, is the exception and will keep for at least two years. A few oils will improve with age, rather like some good wines; examples of these are sandalwood, frankincense, rose otto and patchouli. In fact, a 20-year-old patchouli essence will be extremely mellow and fragrant, and there is even a market for vintage frankincense! Many of the absolutes and resinoids improve with age too, especially jasmine and oak moss.

However, the more often you open the bottle of any aromatic oil, the greater the chance of oxidation and thus of reduction in the oil's therapeutic properties and the quality of its aroma. However, if stored carefully in a cool dark place, they will keep for *at least* one year, from one harvest to the next, with no problem. You should ideally keep your oils in a sealed container and store them in the bottom of the fridge or in a cool larder. If you have a large selection of oils, store them in an old fridge kept for this purpose.

Storage and shelf life of aromatic blends

Once diluted in vegetable oil for use as a massage oil, essential oils will keep for no longer than two months (three if kept in a cool place). Blended into perfumes, your creations will keep for at least six months (or longer if diluted in alcohol). This is because the concentration of essential oils in perfume blends is much higher, while aromatic waters and colognes contain a much lower concentration of essential oils and should be used within three months. You will find that the aroma gradually fades with time, depending on how often the bottle is opened.

Even if you have poured your aromatic creation into a beautiful bottle, do not be tempted to display it on the dressing table near a sunny window — bright light is the number one enemy of essential oils. Do not leave it in the bathroom either as heat and steam will trigger the deterioration of any aromatic product. It is best to make only a small quantity of perfume or aromatic water at a time. Keep it in a drawer or in a cupboard well away from any source of heat, and use it often.

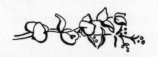

3 Aromatic Profiles

The aromatic oils listed here are those commonly used in perfumery as well as aromatherapy. A great many of the oils can be purchased from health shops and herbal suppliers. However, certain more expensive aromatics, such as mimosa, orange flower absolute, rose otto and carnation, can only be obtained by mail order (see Useful Addresses page 128).

The aromatic oils

Angelica (*Angelica archangelica*)

Source: The essential oil is obtained by steam distillation of roots or the seed from the plant which is native to Europe and Siberia.

Aromatherapy uses: Psoriasis, arthritis, rheumatism, respiratory ailments, fatigue, nervous tension, colds and flu.

Description and odour effect: The root oil is colourless, turning yellow and then dark yellow as it ages. It has a rich herbaceous-earthy scent. The seed oil is colourless and has a fresher, spicy top note. The odour effect of both oils is stimulating and aphrodisiac.

Blends well with: Citrus essences, clary sage, oakmoss, patchouli, vetiver.

CAUTION: The root oil (not the seed oil) should not be applied to the skin shortly before exposure to sunlight as it may cause pigmentation. Avoid during pregnancy.

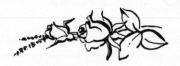

Basil, French (*Ocimum basilicum*)

Source: Steam distillation of the leaves and flowering tops from the herb, native to southern Asia and the Middle East. The oil-producing plants are cultivated throughout Europe.

Aromatherapy uses: Muscular aches and pains, respiratory disorders, scanty menstruation, colds and flu, mental fatigue, anxiety and depression.

Description and odour effect: A colourless or pale yellow liquid with a light, fresh, sweet-spicy scent and balsamic undertone. Its odour effect is at first stimulating, giving way to a warm, comforting feeling.

Blends well with: Bergamot, clary sage, frankincense, geranium, lime, neroli, oakmoss.

CAUTION: Avoid during pregnancy; not to be used on sensitive skin; use in the lowest concentrations. Despite the popularity of basil essence, it is not an oil that I find appealing. Moreover, I believe it should only be used as a room scent due to its potentially irritant effect.

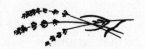

Bergamot (*Citrus bergamia*)

Source: Obtained by expression of the rind of the small orange-like fruit native to Italy.

Aromatherapy uses: Colds and flu, fever, infectious illness, tonsillitis (a few drops in water to be used as a gargle), anxiety, depression.

Description and odour effect: A light green essence with a delightfully citrus aroma with a hint of spice. Refreshing and uplifting to the emotions.

Blends well with: Other citrus essences, basil, clary sage, coriander, cypress, elemi, frankincense, geranium, ginger, lavender, neroli.

CAUTION: Not to be used on the skin shortly before exposure to sunlight as it may cause pigmentation. However, for skin perfumes try to obtain rectified bergamot oil called 'Bergamot FCF', which is free of bergaptene (the substance which causes skin pigmentation). However, whole bergamot oil can be used as a room scent.

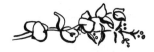

Black Pepper (*Piper nigrum*)

Source: Steam distillation of the dried peppercorns from a woody vine native to south west India. Most of the oil is produced in India, although it is also distilled in Europe and the USA from the imported peppercorns.

Aromatherapy uses: Poor circulation, muscular aches and pains, loss of appetite, nausea, colds and flu, infections and viruses, lethargy, mental fatigue.

Description and odour effect: A pale, greenish-yellow liquid with a hot, spicy, piquant odour. The smell is stimulating and warming; a reputed aphrodisiac.

Blends well with: Other spices, citrus essences, jasmine, lavender, rose, rosemary, sandalwood.

CAUTION: Use in low concentration; avoid if you have sensitive skin.

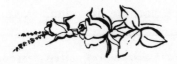

Cardamom (*Elettaria cardamomum*)

Source: Steam distillation of the dried ripe fruit (seeds) from the reed-like herb native to Asia.

Aromatherapy uses: Digestive disturbances, mental fatigue, nervous exhaustion.

Description and odour effect: A colourless to yellowish liquid with a sweet-spicy, warming fragrance. The odour effect is warming and stimulating; a reputed aphrodisiac.

Blends well with: Cedarwood, cinnamon, citrus essences, cloves, floral essences, frankincense.

CAUTION: Use in the lowest concentration as it has a high odour intensity.

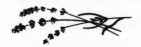

Carnation (*Dianthus carophyllus*)

At the time of writing, although carnation is widely employed in high class perfumery, it is not generally used in aromatherapy. Information on its therapeutic properties is therefore unavailable.

Source: Carnation is mainly cultivated in Egypt to satisfy the demands of the perfume industry. The oil is extracted by volatile solvents, therefore it is an absolute rather than a true essential oil.

Description and odour effect: A light amber-coloured liquid with a mellow, sweet-floral fragrance which also has a spicy kick. The fragrance is extremely tenacious, especially when applied to hair or clothing. Its odour effect is warming and uplifting; a reputed aphrodisiac.

Blends well with: Cedarwood, citrus essences, clary sage, coriander, frankincense, ginger.

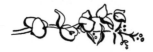

Cedarwood, Atlas (*Cedrus atlantica*)

Source: Steam distillation of the wood, stumps and sawdust from the evergreen tree native to the Atlas Mountains of Algeria, though most of the oil is produced in Morocco.

Aromatherapy uses: Acne, eczema, psoriasis, oily skin, hair loss, dandruff, arthritis, rheumatism, respiratory disorders, cystitis, PMS, nervous tension and stress-related disorders.

Description and odour effect: A dark amber liquid with a warm, camphoraceous top note and a sweet-woody under-tone. The fragrance improves as the oil ages. Its odour effect is sedative and antidepressant; a reputed aphrodisiac.

Blends well with: Bergamot, carnation, clary sage, cypress, frankincense, jasmine, juniper, neroli, rose, rosemary, vetiver, ylang ylang.

CAUTION: Not to be used during pregnancy.

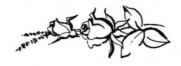

Chamomile, Roman (*Anthemis nobilis*)

Source: Steam distillation of the white, daisy-like flower heads. Native to southern and western Europe.

Aromatherapy uses: Acne, allergies, eczema, inflamed skin conditions, earache, wounds, burns, menstrual problems, PMS, headache, insomnia, nervous tension and stress-related conditions.

Description and odour effect: A pale yellow liquid with a dry, yet sweet-herbaceous aroma. Its odour effect is sedative.

Blends well with: Bergamot, clary sage, geranium, jasmine, lavender, lemon, neroli, oakmoss, rose, ylang ylang.

CAUTION: Use in the lowest concentrations as it has a high odour intensity.

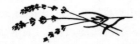

Cinnamon Bark (*Cinnamomum zeylanicum*)

Source: Steam distillation of the bark chips from the small tree native to Sri Lanka, India and Madagascar. A lower grade oil is obtained from the leaves and twigs.

Aromatherapy uses: Used in the vaporizer as an anti-depressant room scent or as an antibiotic, antiviral fumigant during infectious illness.

Description and odour effect: A light amber liquid with a sweet, warm-spicy, dry, tenacious aroma. The odour effect is stimulating and warming; a reputed aphrodisiac.

Blends well with: Citrus essences, frankincense, other spices.

CAUTION: This oil is a powerful skin irritant. Use only as a room scent. Alternatively, you could prepare a decoction from a piece of cinnamon stick which can be vaporized as an environmental fragrance (see Chapter 6).

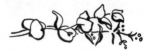

Clary Sage (*Salvia sclarea*)

Source: Steam distillation of the flowering tops and leaves of the oranamental plant which is related to common sage. Native to the Mediterranean region.

Aromatherapy uses: High blood pressure, muscular aches and pains, respiratory problems, menstrual problems, PMS, depression, migraine, nervous tension and stress-related disorders.

Description and odour effect: A colourless or pale yellow liquid with a sweet, herbaceous-floral scent, not at all like common sage. Its odour effect is uplifting and relaxing; a reputed aphrodisiac.

Blends well with: Most oils, especially bergamot, coriander, frankincense, geranium, jasmine, juniper, lavender, oakmoss, pine, vetiver.

CAUTION: Not to be used during pregnancy.

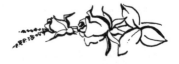

Clove Bud (*Eugenia caryophyllus*)

Source: Water distillation from the buds of the slender evergreen tree native to Indonesia. Most supplies of the oil are from Madagascar. Lower grades of clove oil are distilled from the leaves and stems.

Aromatherapy uses: Vaporized as a room scent, or used as a fumigant during infectious illness. It is also employed as a first aid measure for toothache (the oil is analgesic), but should never be used long-term as it is a skin irritant and will damage the gums. Whilst awaiting dental treatment, a single drop of the oil can be dropped into the tooth cavity or rubbed into the gums.

Description and odour effect: A light amber liquid with a bitter-sweet spicy aroma. The odour effect is warming and stimulating. A reputed aphrodisiac.

Blends well with: Citrus essences, lavender, rose, vanilla, ylang ylang and other spices.

CAUTION: The oil is a powerful skin irritant, so use only as a room scent. Alternatively, prepare a decoction from whole cloves for a vaporizer to perfume rooms (see Chapter 6). Use in the lowest concentration as it has a high odour intensity.

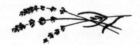

Coriander (*Coriandrum sativum*)

Source: Steam distillation of the herb native to Europe and western Asia. Most of the oil is produced in eastern Europe.

Aromatherapy uses: Arthritis, muscular aches and pains, poor circulation, digestive problems, colds and flu, mental fatigue, nervous exhaustion.

Description and odour effect: A colourless to pale yellow liquid with a sweet, spicy, faintly musky aroma. A stimulating, warming aroma; a reputed aphrodisiac.

Blends well with: Other spices, citrus essences, cypress, frankincense, jasmine, juniper, petitgrain, pine, sandalwood.

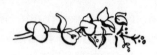

Cypress (*Cupressus sempervirens*)

Source: Steam distillation of the needles, twigs and cones of the tall conifer tree native to the eastern Mediterranean region. Most of the oil is produced in France, Spain and Morocco.

Aromatherapy uses: Oily skin conditions, haemorrhoids, excessive perspiration, gum disorders, varicose veins, wounds, respiratory disorders, circulatory problems, fluid retention, cellulite, rheumatic complaints, excessive menstruation, menopausal problems, nervous tension and stress.

Description and odour effect: A pale yellow liquid with a woody-balsamic odour. Its odour effect is cooling and calming.

Blends well with: Bergamot and other citrus oils, clary sage, juniper, lavender, marjoram, pine, sandalwood.

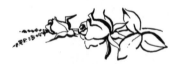

Elemi (*Canarium luzonicum*)

Source: Steam distillation of the gum exudes from the tall tree native to the Philippines and the Moluccas.

Aromatherapy uses: Rheumatic conditions, respiratory disorders, skin infections, nervous exhaustion.

Description and odour effect: A pale yellow or colourless liquid with a strong, spicy-balsamic aroma which also has a citrus-geranium note. The odour effect is tenacious, stimulating and warming.

Blends well with: Citrus essences, cinnamon, clove, coriander, frankincense, lavender, myrrh, rosemary.

CAUTION: Use in the lowest concentration as it has a high odour intensity.

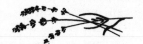

Eucalyptus (*Eucalyptus globulus*)

Source: Steam distillation of the twigs and leaves of the tall evergreen tree native to Australia. Most of the oil is produced from cultivated trees grown in Spain and Portugal.

Aromatherapy uses: Skin infections and wounds, muscular aches and pains, respiratory disorders, cystitis, colds and flu, debility, headaches, neuralgia, mental fatigue.

Description and odour effect: A colourless liquid with a camphoraceous-menthol aroma. The odour is mentally stimulating and cooling.

Blends well with: Cedarwood, cypress, lavender, lemon, marjoram, pine, rosemary.

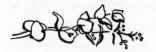

Fennel, Sweet (*Foeniculum vulgare*)

Source: Steam distillation of the crushed seeds from the herb native to the Mediterranean region. Most of the oil is produced in Hungary, Bulgaria, Germany, France, Italy and Greece.

Aromatherapy uses: Bruises, cellulite, fluid retention, constipation, loss of appetite, flatulence, insufficient milk in nursing mothers, menopausal problems.

Description and odour effect: A colourless to pale yellow liquid with a sweet anise-like aroma. The odour effect is warming and stimulating.

Blends well with: Geranium, lavender, sandalwood.

CAUTION: The oil can irritate the skin, especially when used in the bath, so it is best to use it as a room scent only. Avoid during pregnancy. There is also a remote chance that fennel will promote an epileptic seizure, but only in prone subjects. Therefore, avoid if you suffer from epilepsy. The oil has an intense odour, so use in small quantities.

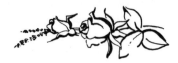

Frankincense (*Boswellia carteri*)

Source: Steam distillation of the gum exudes of the small tree native to north-east Africa.

Aromatherapy uses: Skin care (particularly mature skin), scars, wounds, respiratory ailments, cystitis, colds and flu, anxiety and stress, meditation aid.

Description and odour effect: A colourless to pale yellow liquid with a warm, balsamic fragrance, subtly lemony, and sometimes with a note of camphor. The odour improves greatly as the oil ages. The odour effect is warming and balancing to the emotions.

Blends well with: Cedarwood, cinnamon and other spices, citrus essences, floral essences, sandalwood, vetiver.

Galbanum (*Ferula galbaniflua*)

Source: Water or steam distillation of the gum exudes of the large herb native to the Middle East and western Asia.

Aromatherapy uses: Abscesses, acne, scars, wounds, inflamed skin, poor circulation, muscular aches and pains, rheumatism, respiratory ailments, nervous tension and stress-related disorders.

Description and odour effect: An amber-coloured liquid, becoming viscous as it ages, with a green-woody scent and soft balsamic undertone. The odour effect is calming; a reputed aphrodisiac.

Blends well with: Geranium, lavender, oakmoss, pine, ylang ylang.

CAUTION: Not to be used during pregnancy. The oil has an intense odour, so use in low concentration.

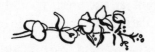

Geranium (*Pelargonium graveolens*)

Source: Steam distillation of the leaves, stalks and flowers of the shrub native to South Africa. Most of the oil is produced in Réunion (Bourbon) and Egypt.

Aromatherapy uses: Skin care, congested skin conditions, dermatitis, eczema, burns, head lice, ringworm, wounds, cellulite, poor circulation, PMS, menopausal symptoms, nervous tension and stress-related conditions.

Description and odour effect: A greenish liquid with a piercingly sweet rose-like scent. Its odour effect is uplifting, but can be highly stimulating to certain individuals, especially young children.

Blends well with: Bergamot and other citrus essences, clary sage, clove, jasmine, juniper, lavender, neroli, patchouli, sandalwood.

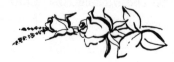

Ginger (*Zingiber officinale*)

Source: Steam distillation of the unpeeled, dried, ground root (rhizomes) of the plant native to southern Asia.

Aromatherapy uses: Arthritis, muscular aches and pains, poor circulation, rheumatism, catarrh, coughs, sore throats, diarrhoea, colic, indigestion, nausea, travel sickness, colds and flu, debility, nervous exhaustion.

Description and odour effect: A pale yellow or amber liquid with a warm, peppery-spicy scent, but in my opinion, not as pleasantly pungent as the fresh root. Its odour effect is warming and stimulating; a reputed aphrodisiac.

Blends well with: Cedarwood, citrus essences, coriander, frankincense, neroli, patchouli, rose, sandalwood, vetiver.

CAUTION: Use in minute quantities as the intense aroma may overpower your blends.

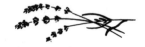

Grapefruit (*Citrus* × *paradisi*)

Source: Expression of the fresh peel of the fruit from a small evergreen tree native to tropical Asia. A lower grade oil with a less attractive odour is obtained by steam distillation of the peel and fruit pulp. The oil is mainly produced in California.

Aromatherapy uses: Cellulite, muscle fatigue, fluid retention, chills, colds and flu, depression, nervous exhaustion.

Description and odour effect: The expressed oil (not the lower grade extraction) is a yellow-green liquid with a fresh, sweet citrus fragrance. Its odour effect is uplifting and anti-depressant.

Blends well with: Other citrus essences, cardamom, coriander, cypress, geranium, lavender, neroli, palmarosa, rosemary.

CAUTION: Do not apply to the skin shortly before exposure to sunlight as it may cause pigmentation.

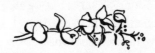

Jasmine (*Jasminum officinale*)

Source: Solvent extraction of the night-scented flowers of the evergreen climber native to China, northern India and western Asia. Most of the oil is produced in Egypt and France.

Aromatherapy uses: Depression, nervous exhaustion and stress-related conditions.

Description and odour effect: The absolute is dark amber and slightly viscous with a warm, floral scent and musky undertone. The fragrance improves as the oil ages. The odour effect is warming, uplifting and a reputed aphrodisiac.

Blends well with: Other florals, citrus essences, clary sage, sandalwood.

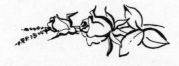

Juniper (*Juniperus communis*)

Source: Steam distillation of the berries of the evergreen shrub native to the northern hemisphere. A lower grade oil with a harsh aroma is extracted from the needles and wood. Always use juniper *berry* oil for perfumery and aromatherapy.

Aromatherapy uses: Acne, eczema, oily skin conditions, cellulite, hair loss, haemorrhoids, rheumatism, colds and flu, absence of periods outside pregnancy, cystitis, anxiety, nervous tension and stress-related problems.

Description and odour effect: A colourless liquid with a fresh, woody aroma reminiscent of pine but with a peppery kick. Its odour effect is warming and calming.

Blends well with: Citrus essences, especially bergamot, cypress, elemi, galbanum, geranium, lavender, oakmoss, pine, rosemary, sandalwood.

CAUTION: Not to be used in pregnancy.

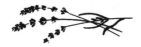

Lavender (*Lavandula angustifolia*)

Source: Steam distillation of the fresh flowering tops of the shrub native to the Mediterranean region.

Aromatherapy uses: Skin care (suits all skin types), acne, athlete's foot, burns, earache, inflammations, insect bites and stings, insect repellent, dandruff, head lice, psoriasis, ringworm, scabies, sunburn, wounds, respiratory ailments, cystitis, PMS, colds and flu, depression, headache, stress-related conditions.

Description and odour effect: A colourless to pale yellow

liquid with a sweet, floral-herbaceous aroma. The odour effect is calming, uplifting and refreshing.

Blends well with: Most oils, especially citrus and floral.

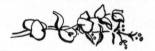

Lemon (*Citrus limonum*)

Source: Expression of the outer part of the fresh peel of the fruit of the small evergreen tree native to Asia and eastern India. Most of the oil is produced in the Mediterranean region, especially Spain and Portugal.

Aromatherapy uses: Oily skin conditions, arthritis, cellulite, high blood pressure, poor circulation, rheumatism, respiratory disorders, colds and flu, depression.

Description and odour effect: A pale yellow-green liquid with a sharp, fresh citrus scent. Try to use within one year of purchase as the aroma rapidly deteriorates with age. Its odour effect is uplifting and refreshing.

Blends well with: Other citrus essences, all florals, eucalyptus, frankincense, juniper, oakmoss.

CAUTION: Do not apply to the skin shortly before exposure to sunlight as it may cause pigmentation.

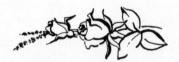

Lime (*Citrus aurantifolia*)

Source: Expression of the peel of the unripe fruit of the small evergreen tree native to southern Asia. There is also a distilled oil which is captured from the whole ripe crushed fruit. Most of the oil is produced in Florida, Cuba, Mexico and Italy.

Aromatherapy uses: Cellulite, poor circulation, respiratory disorders, colds and flu, depression.

Description and odour effect: A pale yellow or green liquid with a fresh, citrus aroma. Try to use within one year of purchase as the aroma rapidly deteriorates with age. The odour effect is uplifting and refreshing.

Blends well with: Other citrus essences, clary sage, lavender, neroli, rosemary, ylang ylang.

CAUTION: The expressed oil can cause unsightly blotching of the skin if applied shortly before exposure to sunlight, but the distilled oil is benign in this respect. However, the aroma of the expressed oil is superior. Use in minute quantities as the aroma may overpower your blends.

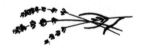

Mandarin (*Citrus reticulata*)

Source: Expression of the peel of the fruit of the small evergreen tree native to southern China and the Far East. Most of the oil is produced in Italy, Spain, Cyprus and Greece.

Aromatherapy uses: Stretch marks, cellulite, fluid retention, digestive problems, insomnia, nervous tension.

Description and odour effect: A yellowy-orange liquid with an intensely sweet citrus aroma. Try to use within one year of purchase as the aroma rapidly deteriorates with age. Its odour effect is soothing and uplifting.

Blends well with: Other citrus essences, neroli, spice oils.

CAUTION: Do not apply to the skin shortly before exposure to sunlight as it may cause pigmentation.

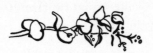

Marjoram (*Origanum marjorana*)

Source: Steam distillation of the dried flowers of the bushy herb native to the Mediterranean region, Egypt and North Africa. Most of the oil is produced in France, Morocco, Egypt and Germany.

Aromatherapy uses: Chilblains, bruises, arthritis, muscular aches and pains, rheumatism, respiratory disorders, colic, constipation, absence of menstruation outside pregnancy, painful menstruation, PMS, colds and flu, insomnia, migraine, nervous tension.

Description and odour effect: A pale yellow liquid with a warm spicy-camphoraceous aroma. Its odour effect is warming and calming and is reputed to quell sexual desire.

Blends well with: Bergamot, cedarwood, chamomile, cypress, eucalyptus, lavender, rosemary.

CAUTION: Not to be used during pregnancy.

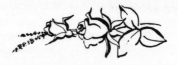

Mimosa (*Acacia dealbata*)

Source: Solvent extraction of the flowers and twig ends of the bushy plant native to Europe and Asia.

Aromatherapy uses: Nervous exhaustion and stress.

Description and odour effect: An amber-coloured viscous

liquid with a light, dry, woody-floral scent vaguely reminiscent of violets. Its odour effect is calming.

Blends well with: Coriander, lavender, neroli, oakmoss, rose, sandalwood, ylang ylang.

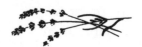

Myrrh (*Commiphora myrrha*)

Source: Steam distillation of the gum of the small tree native to north-east Africa and south-west Asia. A solvent-extracted resinoid is also available, but this is not recommended for home use as it is solid at room temperature and therefore difficult to use.

Aromatherapy uses: Athlete's foot, skin care (especially mature skins), ringworm, wounds, arthritis, respiratory disorders, gum infections, mouth ulcers, absence of menstruation outside pregnancy, thrush, nervous tension.

Description and odour effect: The essential oil is a light amber viscous liquid with a warm, balsamic odour which improves as the oil ages. Its odour effect is warming and relaxing.

Blends well with: Citrus essences, cypress, frankincense, geranium, juniper, lavender, oakmoss, patchouli, pine, sandalwood, spice essences.

CAUTION: Not to be used during pregnancy.

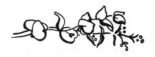

Neroli (*Citrus aurantium var amara*)

Source: Steam distillation of the freshly picked blossom of the bitter orange tree: a small evergreen specimen native to the Far East. A solvent extraction is also available and is known as Orange Flower Absolute. Orange flower water is also produced as by-product of the distillation process. Most of the oil is produced in Italy, Morocco and Egypt.

Aromatherapy uses: Both the essential oil and the absolute can be used for skin care (most skin types), stretch marks, palpitations, poor circulation, diarrhoea, anxiety, depression, PMS, shock and stress-related disorders.

Description and odour effect: The essential oil is pale yellow liquid with a sweet, floral fragrance and bitter undertone. The absolute is a dark amber viscous liquid with a fresh, warm, sweet-floral fragrance, very similar to the scent of fresh orange blossom. The aroma effect of both neroli and orange flower absolute is uplifting, calming and anti-depressant; a reputed aphrodisiac.

Blends well with: Chamomile, citrus essences, clary sage, coriander, jasmine, lavender, myrrh, rose, ylang ylang.

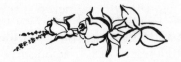

Oakmoss (*Evernia prunastri*)

Source: Solvent extraction of the lichen found growing on oak trees, and sometimes on other species. The lichen is indigenous to Europe and North America.

Aromatherapy uses: Not generally used in aromatherapy, though the oil is said to be antiseptic, demulcent (protects mucous membranes and allays irritation) and expectorant.

Description and odour effect: A dark green, viscous liquid with an extremely tenacious, earthy-mossy odour. The odour improves as the oil ages. Indeed, to my nose, oakmoss needs to be at least 18 months old before it is pleasant to use. Its odour effect is warming and calming.

Blends well with: Most other essences, particularly clary sage, lavender, neroli, petitgrain and rose.

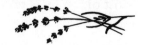

Orange Flower Absolute — see Neroli

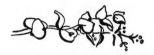

Orange, sweet (*Citrus sinensis*)

Source: Expression of the fresh ripe peel of the fruit of the small evergreen tree native to the Far East. An inferior grade steam distilled oil, obtained from the fruit pulp, is also available. Most of the oil is produced in Italy, Tunisia, Morocco and France.

Aromatherapy uses: Palpitations, fluid retention, respiratory ailments, colds and flu, nervous tension, stress and depression.

Description and odour effect: A pale yellow liquid with a warm, sweet citrus scent. Try to use within one year of purchase as the aroma rapidly deteriorates with age. Its odour effect is uplifting.

Blends well with: Other citrus essences, clary sage, frankincense, lavender, myrrh, neroli, spice oils.

CAUTION: Do not apply to the skin shortly before exposure to sunlight as it may cause pigmentation.

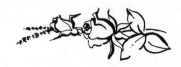

Palmarosa (*Cymbopogon martinii var. martinii*)

Source: Steam or water distillation of the wild grass native to India and Pakistan. Most of the oil is produced in Indonesia, Brazil and the Comoros Islands in the Indian Ocean.

Aromatherapy uses: Acne, minor skin infections, scars, nervous exhaustion.

Description and odour effect: A pale yellow or greenish liquid with a sweet, floral geranium-like scent. Its odour effect is stimulating and uplifting.

Blends well with: Floral essences, cedarwood, geranium, oakmoss, sandalwood.

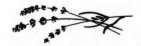

Patchouli (*Pogostemon cablin*)

Source: Steam distillation of the dried leaves of the bushy plant native to tropical Asia. Most of the oil is produced in India, China, Malaysia and South America.

Aromatherapy uses: Acne, athlete's foot, fungal infections, dandruff, insect repellent, wounds, nervous exhaustion and stress-related complaints.

Description and odour effect: An amber, slightly viscous liquid with a rich, earthy scent, becoming sweeter as it ages. The oil ideally needs to be at least two or three years old for perfumery purposes. Its odour effect is warming, stimulating and a reputed aphrodisiac.

Blends well with: Bergamot, cedarwood, clary sage, clove, geranium, lavender, neroli, oakmoss, rose, sandalwood, vetiver.

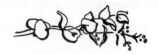

Peppermint (*Mentha piperita*)

Source: Steam distillation of the flowering tops of the herb native to Europe.

Aromatherapy uses: Respiratory disorders, digestive disturbances, colds and flu, fevers, fainting, headache, migraine, mental fatigue.

Description and odour effect: A pale yellow liquid with a piercing minty-camphoraceous odour. Its odour effect is stimulating and cooling.

Blends well with: Eucalyptus, lavender, lemon, marjoram, rosemary.

CAUTION: Use in the lowest concentrations as it may irritate sensitive skin. Too much peppermint will also overpower your blends.

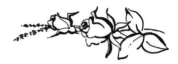

Petitgrain (*Citrus aurantium var. amara*)

Source: Steam distillation of the leaves and twigs of the bitter orange tree native to southern China and north-east India. Most of the oil is produced in France.

Aromatherapy uses: Oily skin conditions, nervous exhaustion and stress-related disorders.

Description and odour effect: A pale yellow liquid with a fresh, woody, bitter-sweet scent reminiscent of neroli, but less refined. Its odour effect is refreshing and uplifting.

Blends well with: Bergamot, clary sage, clove, geranium, jasmine, lavender, neroli, oakmoss, orange flower absolute, palmarosa, rosemary.

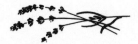

Pine, Scotch (*Pinus sylvestris*)

Source: Dry distillation of the needles of the evergreen tree native to Scotland and Norway. Most of the oil is produced in the eastern USA from cultivated trees.

Aromatherapy uses: Excessive perspiration, arthritis, muscular aches and pains, poor circulation, rheumatism, respiratory ailments, cystitis, colds and flu, fatigue, nervous exhaustion.

Description and odour effect: A colourless to pale yellow liquid with dry-balsamic, turpentine-like aroma. Its odour effect is cooling, mentally stimulating, yet also comforting to the emotions.

Blends well with: Bergamot, cedarwood, eucalyptus, juniper, lavender, lemon, marjoram, rosemary.

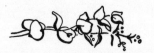

Rose, Cabbage (*Rosa centifolia*)

Source: Solvent extraction of the petals of the flower native to the Middle East. However, most of the oil is produced in Morocco and France from hybrid roses.

Aromatherapy uses: Skin care, thread veins, dry skin, eczema, palpitations, poor circulation, hay fever, irregular menstruation, uterine disorders, depression and stress-related disorders.

Description and odour effect: The absolute is yellowy-orange and slightly viscous with a sweet, mellow, spicy-floral fragrance. Its odour effect is calming, uplifting and anti-depressant. A reputed aphrodisiac.

Blends well with: Most oils, especially sandalwood.

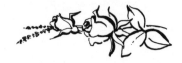

Rose Otto (*Rosa damascena*)

Source: Steam distillation of the petals of the damask rose which is native to the Orient, but now cultivated mainly in Bulgaria. Rosewater is a by-product of the distillation process.

Aromatherapy uses: As for Cabbage Rose.

Description and odour effect: A colourless to pale yellow liquid, semi-solid at room temperature. In order to make the oil liquid, place the bottle in a cup of hand-warm water for about 30 seconds before use. Never use very hot water as this will have a detrimental effect on the oil. The fragrance of the oil is sweet and mellow with a hint of vanilla and clove, extremely tenacious, becoming more mellow as the oil ages. The odour effect is intoxicating, antidepressant and warming. A reputed aphrodisiac.

Blends well with: Most oils, especially citrus essences and sandalwood.

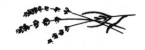

Rosmary (*Rosmarinus officinalis*)

Source: Steam distillation of the fresh, flowering tops of the shrubby evergreen herb native to the Mediterranean region.

The main oil producing countries are France, Spain and Tunisia.

Aromatherapy uses: Dandruff, oily skin and hair conditions, promotes hair growth, head lice, muscular aches and pains, fluid retention, poor circulation, rheumatism, colds and flu, low blood pressure, mental fatigue, nervous exhaustion.

Description and odour effect: A colourless or pale yellow liquid with a piercing, fresh herbaceous scent. Poor quality oils smell camphoraceous, like eucalyptus. Its odour effect is refreshing, and mentally stimulating, but with a warming quality. A reputed aphrodisiac due to its stimulating effect.

Blends well with: Basil, bergamot, cedarwood, cinnamon, coriander, elemi, frankincense, lavender, peppermint, petitgrain, pine.

CAUTION: To be avoided by sufferers of epilepsy — the oil may trigger an attack.

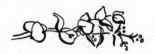

Sandalwood (*Santalum album*)

Source: Water or steam distillation of the roots and heartwood of the small, evergreen tree native to tropical Asia. The best quality oil comes from Mysore in India.

Aromatherapy uses: Acne, dry skin, oily skin, respiratory ailments, nausea, cystitis, depression, insomnia, stress-related disorders.

Description and odour effect: A pale yellow, slightly viscous oil with a warm, soft sweet-woody scent of excellent tenacity. The fragrance improves as the oil ages. The odour effect is calming and antidepressant; a reputed aphrodisiac.

Blends well with: Bergamot, black pepper, clove, fennel, jasmine, lavender, mimosa, oakmoss, patchouli, rose, vetiver.

CAUTION: Not to be confused with West Indian sandalwood or amyris (*Amyris balsamifera*), which is less expensive, but has a very different aroma of poor tenacity.

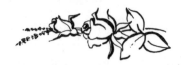

Vanilla (*Vanilla planifolia*)

Source: Solvent extraction of the vanillin crystals which form on the fermented vanilla beans. The plant is an herbaceous climbing orchid native to Mexico, cultivated mainly in Madagascar, Tahiti, Mexico and the Comoros Islands in the Indian Ocean. The absolute is very hard to obtain and extremely expensive when it is available. Therefore, all the vanilla recipes suggested in Chapters 6 and 7 contain the home-made infused oil or a water extraction of the pods.

Aromatherapy uses: Not generally used in aromatherapy, though if the aroma is liked, I employ it as a mood-enhancing room scent (blended with other essences) for those suffering from depressive states of mind.

Description and odour effect: The absolute is a dark brown viscous liquid with a rich, sweet balsamic, vanilla-like (there is no other way to describe it!) fragrance. The odour effect of vanilla is warming, uplifting and comforting; a reputed aphrodisiac.

Blends well with: Clove, lime, neroli, rose, sandalwood, vetiver, ylang ylang.

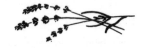

Vetiver (*Vetiveria zizanoides*)

Source: Steam distillation of the roots of the scented grass native to southern India, Indonesia and Sri Lanka. Most of the oil is obtained from cultivated plants grown in Réunion and the Comoros Islands.

Aromatherapy uses: Acne, oily skin conditions, wounds, arthritis, muscular aches and pains, rheumatism, insomnia, nervous tension.

Description and odour effect: A dark brown viscous liquid with a rich, earthy, molasses-like odour. The fragrance improves as the oil ages. Its odour effect is calming and warming; a reputed aphrodisiac.

Blends well with: Clary sage, jasmine, lavender, mimosa, oakmoss, patchouli, rose, sandalwood, ylang ylang.

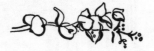

Ylang Ylang (*Cananga odorata var. genuina*)

Source: Water or steam distillation of the flowers of the tall, tropical tree native to Asia. Most of the oil is produced in Madagascar, Réunion and the Comoros Islands. There are four grades of ylang ylang labelled Ylang Ylang Extra, then Ylang Ylang 1, 2 and 3. Always use ylang ylang extra which is the most expensive and has a vastly superior fragrance.

Aromatherapy uses: Promotes hair growth; high blood pressure, palpitations, depression, insomnia, nervous tension, stress-related disorders.

Description and odour effect: A pale yellow liquid with an intensely sweet, floral scent reminiscent of a blend of jasmine and almonds. Its odour effect is intoxicating and antidepressant; a reputed aphrodisiac.

Blends well with: other florals, citrus essences, frankincense, geranium, vetiver.

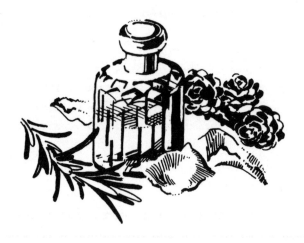

4 The Alchemist's Workshop

The aromatic materials listed in the previous chapter would be extremely costly if you were to go out and buy them all at once. Indeed, my own collection of around 50 essences has developed over a number of years. If you wish to begin experimenting with aromatics, about half a dozen carefully chosen essences are all you need. These will form the basis for a number of interesting fragrant blends and, as you become more familiar with the oils, no doubt you will wish to add to your collection. Here is a guide to the different price ranges of the oils,

Lowest price range: cedarwood, cypress, eucalyptus, fennel, geranium, grapefruit, lavender, lemon, lime, mandarin, marjoram, orange, palmarosa, patchouli, peppermint, petitgrain, pine, rosemary, vetiver.

Medium price range: basil, bergamot, black pepper, cinnamon bark, clary sage, clove bud, coriander, elemi, ginger, juniper berry, myrrh, oakmoss, ylang ylang.

High price range: cardamom, chamomile, frankincense, galbanum, sandalwood.

Very pricy: angelica, carnation, jasmine, mimosa, neroli, orange flower absolute, rose absolute, rose otto, vanilla absolute.

Initially you will be guided by your aroma preference. However, do not be put off by an essence that does not immediately smell interesting. You may discover that it smells wonderful when used in tiny quantities and blended with other essences. Until you have become familiar with the character of each essential oil and have learned to trust your intuition and aromatic good taste, you will just have to take my word for it! Clary sage, for example, has been credited with the power to induce euphoria; but on first acquaintance with its sweet herbaceous aroma, you may be disappointed. However, clary sage is one of the most versatile essences in the perfumier's repertoire. It smells much better in dilution, especially when blended with other essences such as petitgrain, bergamot, rose and ylang ylang. Clary helps to pull together the individual elements of a blend, thus enabling it to resonate as a harmonious whole.

Then there are the tenacious earthy scents of vetiver and patchouli. Blend these with larger quantities of bergamot, lavender or geranium, for instance, and there is a successful marriage of opposites. The brighter citrus or floral notes act to awaken the heavy lingerers, elevating the aroma to a higher plane. At the same time, the powerful embrace of vetiver or patchouli serves to hold back the more volatile essences whose presence would otherwise be relatively fleeting (see Chapter 5).

The art of smelling

No doubt you have already discovered that none of the senses is so easily fatigued as the sense of smell. This is noticed first by an increasing sluggishness, followed by complete odour insensitivity. Therefore, when smelling essential oils, you will have to limit yourself to about half a dozen per session. Similarly, you will only be able to create one perfume at a time, or perhaps two or three if you opt for simple duets. Always work in a well ventilated area which is also moderately warm and free from cooking and other household smells. Undiluted essences are very power-ful and can cause headaches or nausea if inhaled for too long in an overheated or stuffy room.

Choose a time when you are feeling calm and receptive. Ensure that you will not be disturbed for at least 20 minutes – the art of smelling is serious business! Sit in a comfortable position; clear your air passages before you start by breathing rapidly in and out through your nose a few times. Put one drop of the oil (or blend) on to a purpose designed smelling paper (see page 62), or piece of blotting paper. Waft it around in order to encourage vaporization, then inhale the fragrance slowly and deeply, allowing yourself to experience fully its effect.

Stay with the fragrance for a couple of minutes. What does the aroma make you think of? Is it a feeling, memory or image you would like to have more often? On a practical level, would the aroma be suitable as a room scent or a skin perfume? For instance, while peppermint, rosemary and eucalyptus (used singly or blended together) make a refresh-ing environmental fragrance conducive to mental work, not many people would choose to wear these rather medicinal essences as perfume. On the other hand, the velvety scent of sandalwood makes a lovely skin perfume (or a room scent) alone or blended with other essences, especially floral oils. In other words, a successful skin perfume has a sensuous quality rather than a hygienic, deodorizing effect. However, you might find the hygienic-smelling essences suitable for the bath, or blended in minute quantities with more sensuous essences.

This smelling technique can also be used as a form of therapy. Should an aroma make you feel uncomfortable in any way, perhaps evoking an unhappy memory or a disturbing image, it is helping to write about your feelings in depth. It is by viewing an upsetting feeling, memory or image in the sunlight of conscious awareness that it becomes less threatening, perhaps totally disempowered. I have occasionally used this method with willing aromatherapy clients, helping them to work through their distress (often stemming from some half-forgotten childhood trauma), thus enabling the feelings to be released into the present. Of course, positive associations should be recorded too, for this will remind you to include those essences in your mood-enhancing blends. The exercise also serves as a basis for developing and trusting your intuition, which is essential to creative work of any nature.

Perfumery starter selection

Your initial selection of oils will ideally include a represent-ative from each of the eight aroma families listed below. The woody and pine-like families could be grouped together, partly because they are from trees and partly because they tend to blend well with each other, albeit in a rather conservative way. If you are only interested in room scents, a representative from the cheaper herbaceous, pine and citrus families will probably suffice. However, personal perfumes may need to be more sensuous, containing at least one of the expensive florals, according to your aroma preference.

Aromatic families

Balsamic or resinous – elemi, frankincense, galbanum, myrrh, oakmoss.

Citrus – bergamot, grapefruit, lemon, lime, mandarin, orange.

Earthy – angelica, patchouli, vetiver.

Floral – carnation, geranium, jasmine, lavender, mimosa, neroli, orange flower absolute, rose otto, rose absolute, ylang ylang.

Herbaceous – basil, chamomile, clary sage, petitgrain, rosemary.

Pine-like – cypress, juniper, pine.

Spicy – black pepper, cardamom, cinnamon bark, clove, coriander, ginger.

Woody – cedarwood, sandalwood.

CAUTION: Cinnamon and clove should only be used to perfume rooms as these essences can irritate the skin. However, you can make an interesting room scent by preparing a decoction from whole cloves or a piece of cinnamon stick (see Chapter 7).

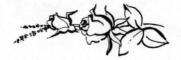

Perfume carriers

Most commercial perfumes and colognes are suspended in alcohol, usually ethanol. Pure alcohol is not generally available in Britain without a perfumier's licence, although in some other countries it can be purchased from pharmacies. Therefore, in order to satisfy those readers who can obtain perfume grade alcohol, I have included instructions for its use in Chapter 6. However, essential oils can be partially suspended in distilled water or in a floral water such as rosewater or orange flower water. The aromatic material will float on the surface so the mixture will need to be poured through a coffee filter paper before use.

Aromatherapists tend to favour oil or beeswax-based perfumes which are much kinder to the skin (alcohol can be very drying for some skins). Oil-based perfumes also have the advantage of lingering on the skin for much longer. However, they do smell a little different from alcoholic or aqueous mixtures, even when they are composed of exactly the same essential oils. Apart from the greater tenacity of oil-based perfumes, the oil itself imparts a sensuous quality to the blend.

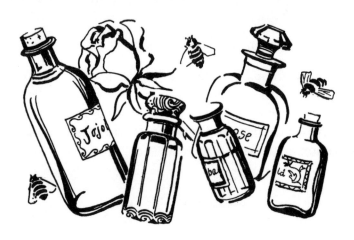

The best base oil for perfumes is jojoba oil (pronounced *ho ho ba*). In fact, jojoba is a virtually odourless liquid wax rather than a true vegetable oil, extracted from a small evergreen plant native to the desert regions of South America. It has a very long shelf-life. Indeed, I have never known the oil turn rancid, which is why it makes an excellent base for perfume. Alternatively, you could use fractionated coconut oil, usually labelled 'Light Coconut', which is a highly refined oil (thus with a long shelf-life) and, unlike whole coconut oil, is not solid at room temperature. Whole coconut oil needs to be melted before you can successfully incorporate the essential oils (place the jar in a cup of hand-hot water for a minute or two). For obvious reasons, if you opt for whole coconut oil as a base, the perfume will need to be stored in a little pot rather than a bottle.

Also included in the aromatic concoctions section is a recipe for making solid perfume. The honey-scented beeswax used in the base imparts its own subtle fragrance to the blend.

Ingredients for making perfume

This is the list of all the ingredients you will need (apart from at least six essential oils) and where they can be obtained:

Alcohol – available from pharmacies in some countries, but not Britain. Ask for perfume grade alcohol, labelled 'ethanol'.

Beeswax – available from herbal suppliers, craft shops or some beekeepers. There are two kinds of beeswax, yellow or white. The latter is a refined version; use whichever you prefer.

Distilled water (de-ionized water) – available from most chemists. Unlike ordinary water, distilled water does not go stale.

Floral waters – orange flower water or rosewater are available from most chemists. However, it is increasingly difficult to obtain real floral waters – the by-products of the distillation process. Unfortunately unscrupulous retailers often sell artificially perfumed products and pass them off for the real thing. If in doubt, order from an essential oil suppliers.

Jojoba – available from health shops or by mail order from essential oil suppliers.

Light coconut oil – available from essential oil suppliers. Whole coconut oil is available from chemists.

Optional extras

Almond oil (or other high quality vegetable oil) – should you wish to make aromatherapy massage oils, almond is one of the finest bases in which to dilute the essential oils. Other recommended base oils include grapeseed and sunflower. For facial treatments, you may wish to use one of the speciality oils such as jojoba, peach kernel, apricot kernel or avocado. Avocado is an excellent oil for very dry skin, but could be made less rich by diluting it 50/50 (or less) with any other base oil if desired. These oils are available from health shops, a few chemists or by mail order from essential oil suppliers.

Smelling strips – for smelling tests. These are absorbent strips of paper 5mm–1 cm (¼–½ inch) wide, and at least 10 cm (4 inches) long to allow sufficient space between the hand and the nose. Alternatively, use blotting paper cut into strips of a similar size, or a damp cotton wool bud.

Vanilla pod – for making your own vanilla extracts. Available from delicatessens, wholefood shops or herbal suppliers.

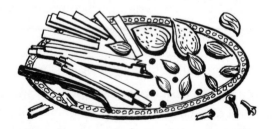

Whole spices – cloves, nutmeg, cinnamon stick, coriander, cardamom. These can be infused in water and used in the essential oil vaporizer as room scents.

Equipment

Screw-top bottles and jars — these are available in various sizes from most chemists and essential oil suppliers, or from specialist shops selling home-made cosmetic materials and herbs. You can, of course, re-cycle any suitable glass containers, but do not use plastic bottles and jars. Essential oils tend to react with plastic, especially if in contact with the substance for any length of time. If you can obtain a glass atomizer (a perfume spray bottle) from a chemist, this would be ideal for an aromatic water or cologne.

Other useful items include:

Essential oil burner or electric fragrancer — for vaporizing essences in the home. These are widely available from health shops, craft outlets and by mail order from essential oil suppliers.

Coffee filter paper — for filtering aromatic waters.

Eye dropper or pipette

Glass measuring jug

Small funnel

Heat-resistant glass or pottery bowl — to fit over a small saucepan of simmering water (the bain-marie method) for making solid perfumes.

Kitchen grater — suitable for grating beeswax.

Fine muslin or fine mesh tea strainer — for straining infusions of whole spices.

Plastic 5 ml medicine spoon — for measuring small quantities of base oil (available from chemists).

Self-adhesive labels — for labelling your aromatic concoctions.

Spirit pen – this has smudge-proof ink, ideal for labelling aromatic concoctions. Available from most stationers.

Notebook – for recording the formulae of your own aromatic masterpieces. There is nothing more frustrating than creating a lovely fragrance and not being able to reproduce it. It would also be useful to record your failures, too – it is surprisingly easy to find yourself making the same discordant mixtures over and over again.

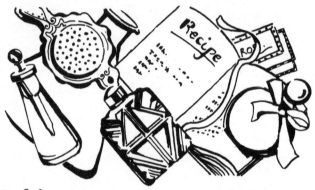

Useful measures

All quantities for the aromatic concoctions in chapters 6 and 7 are given in metric measures. However, it is useful to know approximate conversions.

Liquid measurements

5 ml = 1 teaspoon
10 ml = 1 dessertspoon
15 ml = 1 tablespoon

When measuring essential oils, approximately:

20 drops = 1 ml essential oil
40 drops = 2 ml essential oil
60 drops = 3 ml essential oil
etc

American measurements are slightly different. Approximate conversions are:

2 tablespoons = 1 fluid oz = 30 ml
1 cup = 3 fluid oz = 240 ml
2 cups = 1 pint = 480 ml

Weight

Approximately:

1 oz = 28 g
1 lb = 454 g

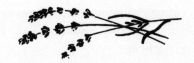

5 Creative Blending

Creating perfume is like painting a beautiful landscape or composing music. The base of the perfume corresponds to the main theme; other essences in the blend are the colours or sounds which add interest and contrast, combining to form a harmonious whole.

It was the nineteenth-century French perfumier Piesse who first classified odours according to the notes in the musical scale. His vision continues to inspire perfumiers and aromatherapists alike, for essential oils are still divided into 'top', 'middle' and 'base' notes.

The top notes of a perfume are highly volatile which means they do not last long. These are essences such as bergamot, lemon and coriander. They form the scent's first impression, giving brightness and clarity to the blend, much as the flute adds high-pitched purity to an orchestra. The middle or 'heart' notes last a little longer; they impart warmth and fullness to the perfume. Rose, clary sage and ylang ylang are some of the most popular middle notes. Then there are the heavier-smelling, deeply resonating base notes which have a profound influence on the blend as a whole: oakmoss, patchouli, vetiver and sandalwood. They are very long-lasting and at the same time 'fix' other essences. This means they slow down the volatility rate of the top and middle notes, thus improving on the tenacity of the perfume as a whole.

Some essential oils are good 'bridges' – they resonate from more than one level, connecting individual components and allowing them to blend. Although not always classified as 'fixatives' in the general sense (i.e. heavy-smelling and tenacious), they slow down the evaporation rate of essences resonating from a slightly higher plane. Bergamot, for example, though highly volatile itself, tempers the evaporation rate of the even flightier lemon or grapefruit. Neroli, a heart note, has the same action on bergamot oil. A good bridging essence also has the ability to awaken the more receptive elements of the heavier aromas. The deeply resonating scents of vetiver, patchouli and jasmine, for instance, can be elevated by the presence of lavender, clary sage, or bergamot.

Adapting perfumes

If you have composed a perfume that smells too garish, with the top note being far removed from the heart note, you can bring the formula into harmony by adding an essence with a softer quality that at the same time vibrates from the middle towards the upper sphere. Rose otto or clary sage would be a good choice.

If, on the other hand, the base note has become too pronounced, having no connection with the heart, you will need to lift the aroma by adding an essence that smells a little brighter, resonating from middle to base: carnation or ylang ylang, for instance.

Should the base note still be predominant, continue to build the perfume by adding a drop or two of a lighter or fresher-smelling essence, one that resonates from middle to top: lavender or geranium.

Of course, your perfumes need not be so complex:

oakmoss (base), lavender (middle) and bergamot (top) would together make a lovely blend with a feeling of green woods and dappled sunlight, the bergamot adding the warm tinge. Alternatively, you may decide to use all top notes in a blend: a traditional eau de cologne mixture perhaps, composed mainly of citrus oils, or a blend composed entirely of middle notes, or of base notes — or whatever permutation you can think of. However, should you opt for all top notes, do not expect the fragrance to be anything more than a brief encounter, as it is the base notes which give perfumes a longer life.

You may also discover that a certain essence radiates a special synergy, the individual elements of its make-up in perfect accord. Such an essence can be used as a perfume all by itself — after all, why blend when you don't have to? Rose otto and carnation are beautiful as perfumes in their own right. Or you might find jasmine, ylang ylang, patchouli or sandalwood attractive as loners.

Perfume notes

The following list categorizes all the essential oils and absolutes profiled in Chapter 3 (plus a few others) according to their perfume notes. Remember that individual essences resonate mainly from the top, middle or base, but at the same time, many are composed of elements that reach up (or down) to an adjacent sphere. As explained, these make good bridges. However, rose essence could be described as the bridging note supreme, for although resonating mainly from the heart, it also embraces both head and base. Indeed, at one time no perfume (whether regarded as a feminine or a masculine fragrance) was deemed complete without the inclusion of rose. Two other oils which enhance just about any perfume are oakmoss and lavender.

Top notes

Angelica	Eucalyptus	Lime
Basil	Fennel	Mandarin
Bergamot	Grapefruit	Orange
Cardamom	Lavender	Peppermint
Coriander	Lemongrass	Petitgrain

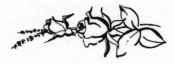

Top to middle

Angelica	Fennel	Neroli
Basil	Geranium	Petitgrain
Bergamot	Lavender	Tagetes
Cardamom	Lemongrass	

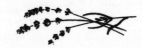

Middle to top

Black pepper	Galbanum	Palmarosa
Chamomile	Geranium	Pine needle
Clary sage	Juniper	Rose absolute
Clove (*room scent*)	Lavender	Rose otto
	Neroli	

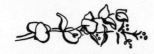

Middle notes

Black pepper	Clary sage	Galbanum
Cinnamon bark (*room scent*)	Clove (*room scent*)	Geranium
		Ginger

Juniper
Lavender
Marjoram
Mimosa
Neroli

Orange flower
  absolute
Palmarosa
Pine needle
Rose absolute

Rose otto
Rosemary
Vanilla
Ylang ylang

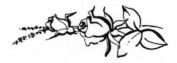

Middle to base

Carnation
Cypress
Jasmine

Myrrh
Orange flower
  absolute

Rose otto
Vanilla
Ylang ylang

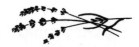

Base to middle

Cedarwood
Elemi
Frankincense
Jasmine

Myrrh
Oakmoss
Sandalwood

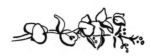

Base notes

Cedarwood
Frankincense
Oakmoss

Patchouli
Sandalwood
Vetiver

Odour effects

Essential oils and other aromatics have been classified according to their perceived effect upon mood: erogenic (or arousing), narcotic (or intoxicating), anti-erogenic (or refreshing), stimulating. Of course, it is important to like the aroma for it to exert its mood-enhancing effect. Unlike mind-bending drugs, essential oils can only work their gentle magic if we are open and receptive to their charms. If we dislike a particular fragrance it will have no effect — unless, of course, we dislike it intensely enough to elicit a gut-felt 'ugh!'.

Erogenic (sex stimulating) — oils which have an obviously 'animal' quality, reminiscent of bodily odours — costus root, musk seed. Also oils which have an erogenic component as part of their chemical make-up, but which few people can detect on a conscious level — neroli, rose.

Narcotic (intoxicating) — the fragrances of flowers, resins and balsams which could be described as sweet or mellow — benzoin, carnation, frankincense, hyacinth, jasmine, narcissus, neroli (to a degree), orange flower absolute, rose, tuberose, vanilla, violet, ylang ylang. These oils tend to dull the keenness of our logical thought processes (left brain activity), so that our perceptions become less distinct and more intuitive (right brain activity), thus engendering a sense of relaxation and openness to other influences. However, in high concentration the narcotic florals tend to cause headaches and sometimes slight nausea. Incidentally, the scent of natural narcotic drugs such as opium smoke and cannabis resin also have this sweet, mellow fragrance.

Anti-erogenic (refreshing) — terpene and camphoraceous odours which could be described as acidic, sharp, or cooling — bergamot, camphor, eucalyptus, lavender, lemon, lemongrass, lime, pine, rosemary (only the lower grade oil which is eucalyptus-like).

Stimulating (activating, exciting): spicy, bitter or menthol − black pepper, clove, cinnamon, coriander, eucalyptus, ginger, peppermint, rosemary.

As you can see, certain odours belong to more than one group, a reflection of the multifarious nature of their chemical make-up. This is especially noticeable with blends of essences. For example, honey-like odours, combining a sweet-floral note with an animal undertone, have a narcotic and an erogenic effect, e.g. a blend of sandalwood and rose. Fruity odours combining an acidic with a sweet odour have a mildly narcotic effect, e.g. a blend of lavender, mandarin and bergamot. Minty odours, which are spicy and camphoraceous at the same time, have an anti-erogenic and a stimulating effect, e.g. a blend of marjoram, basil and peppermint.

Aphrodisiac blends

Many people who wear perfume, cologne or aftershave do so consciously or subconsciously as a means of attraction − as an aphrodisiac. The most successful fragrances in this respect are those which are *subliminally* reminiscent of bodily secretions. The most powerfully erogenic scents are said to be those of animal origin, that is to say, extracted from the sex glands of the musk deer or the civet cat. There is also ambergris, an oily substance of pathological origin which is expelled from the intestines of whales, and is sometimes found floating on the sea. Ambergris is the only odoriferous material of animal origin which is actually pleasant in high concentration. However, apart from the astronomical cost of these substances, the use of animal extractions in perfumery is objectionable to a great many people. However, there are erogenic aromatics of vegetable origin which can be substituted.

There are only two plant oils which have distinct 'animal'

odours, namely costus root and the exorbitantly priced musk seed (ambrette). The oils which I have chosen to feature in this book are the essences which contain *constituents* with erogenic effects. Although some of these constituents are chemically related to those present in the secretions and excretions of the human body, more often they have only similar odours.

As well as oils such as carnation, rose and jasmine, the herbaceous-smelling rosemary essence is, surprisingly, reputed to be an aphrodisiac – as Napoleon discovered through his extravagant use of over sixty bottles of rosemary cologne each month! Many of the balsams and resins such as frankincense, oakmoss, galbanum and vanilla have an erogenic undertone, which can be enhanced by the presence of floral essences or spices (see also the psycho-aromatherapy chart in Chapter 7). However, some of the most beautiful aphrodisiac fragrances are potentially toxic and are therefore not recommended for home use, for instance oils such as narcissus, tonka bean and tuberose.

Considering that valerian essence smells strongly of stale sweat, one would suppose that in high dilution it would be erogenic. However, I have tried using minute quantities of the oil in combination with all manner of sweet essences, but its murky odour always comes through. Maybe you will have better luck.

Rose oil is one of the most interesting of the aphrodisiac oils, for its sweet, mellow fragrance owes much to the mood-altering substance phenylethal alcohol which has both a narcotic and an erogenic effect – the latter is caused by a faint putrid nuance. This substance is a form of PEA (phenylethylamine), a naturally occurring opiate which is produced in the brain when we are in love. Rosewater, a by-product of the distillation process, is higher in phenylethyl alcohol because the substance gives itself more readily to water.

Generally speaking, erogenic essences work equally well

for men and women, their subtle nature being essentially androgynous. Likewise, our sex hormones (and their related pheromones) could also be described as androgynous, as both men and women secrete oestrogen and testosterone, albeit in differing amounts. And while the sex pheromone androstenone is essentially masculine, tiny quantities of this musky odour are also produced by women, contributing to their libido. However, some researchers refute the claim that highly sexed women secrete larger quantities of androstenone.

Blending aphrodisiac oils

When blending the secret is to mix the oils in the correct proportions. Most people would agree that the deeply resonating essences such as sandalwood, vetiver and frankincense harmonize especially well with the masculine body scent. However, the same essences can still form part of a feminine blend if they are kept in the background. Similarly, a subtle floral note would add interest to an essentially masculine fragrance. Of course, aroma preference is the vital guide. The aromas we like best tend to reflect our own body scent as well as our emotional needs. If a woman chooses a heavy vetiver-based perfume, or a man plumps for a predominance of rose, then so be it. The perfume always changes on the skin, becoming something new, at best a fragrance which is in tune with the person's secret instincts.

How aphrodisiac oils work

According to the masters of the old French perfumery schools, an aphrodisiac effect is achieved by an interaction of all the different types of odour effects as already described. Indeed, most modern perfumes also contain components representing all four of the odour-effect groups. But what is the reasoning behind this?

The highly volatile, anti-erogenic top notes of the perfume act to awaken the senses. Although their presence is fleeting, they stimulate interest and susceptibility to the narcotic element of the blend. While this will never act as an aphrodisiac by itself, it will make the user especially receptive to the erogenic sensations received by the other senses — pleasant surroundings, soft music, wonderful food and an attractive companion. The stimulating notes of the perfume have a similar predisposing and preparatory function as the narcotic element. They stimulate the sense of smell so that it reacts to even the faintest odours — to the 'animal' nuance of the blend. The increased receptivity for erogenic odours, triggered by the combination of narcotic and stimulating notes, results in an activation of erotic feelings and images.

Sandalwood, cedarwood and frankincense have been used in the Orient for thousands of years, both as aphrodisiacs and holy incense. This is an example of narcotic and erogenic elements working together, predisposing the individual for meditation or religious ecstasy, rather than the joys of the flesh. It is all a matter of focus — the same type of odours act as aphrodisiacs when applied in different surroundings. Indeed, the divide between religious and sexual ecstasy is tenuous:

> *The pain was so great that I screamed aloud: but simultaneously I felt such infinite sweetness that I wished it to last eternally. It was not bodily but psychic pain, although it affected to a certain extent also the body. It was the sweetest caressing of the soul by God.*

No, not Lady Chatterley, but St Teresa of Avila describing her mystical union with Christ (from her *Life*, written in 1565).

Fragrance and personality

Some perfumiers are of the opinion that our choice of fragrance is non-rational and cannot be explained in psychological terms. Others insist that it is our physique combined with the colour of our hair and eyes that determine which fragrances are right for us. For instance, a tiny blue-eyed blonde woman is told that she should never wear a heavy sultry perfume, which is more suited to a curvaceous black beauty; instead she must opt for a fresh, anti-erogenic scent. Yet the blonde woman's innerself, as expressed through her aroma preference, may well be big and voluptuous!

The majority of perfumiers focus on the relationship between personality and aroma preference: extroverts who need a great deal of stimulation tend towards fresh green scents or sharp fruity fragrances. Introverts are attracted to sweet oriental notes, whereas those who are neither markedly extrovert nor introvert show no significant tendency towards any one specific kind of fragrance note.

It is my own belief that personality plays a part, as do passing moods, state of health and also the time of day and the seasons. Our perception of odour is constantly moving, reflecting the shifting patterns of the bodymind complex.

In Germany, some people who specialize in bespoke fragrances use the colour-rosette test (reproduced opposite in black and white) as a decision-making aid. If you so wish, you can colour in the rosette using the colour keys provided. The customer is asked to look at several different multi-coloured floral patterns displayed around a black circle, and to choose the rosette which appeals to them the most. They also indicate which rosette they find the least attractive. The consultant advises the client not to choose on the basis of which colours they think suit them, or which happen to be in fashion at the time. Also colour harmony should not be a deciding factor (some of the colour combinations would grate on those with a knowledge of graphic art). In other

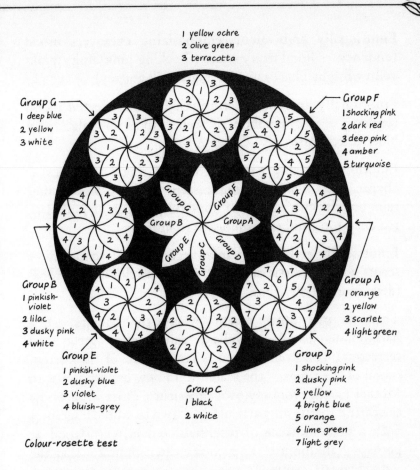

1 yellow ochre
2 olive green
3 terracotta

Group G
1 deep blue
2 yellow
3 white

Group F
1 shocking pink
2 dark red
3 deep pink
4 amber
5 turquoise

Group G Group F
Group B Group A
Group E Group D
Group C

Group A
1 orange
2 yellow
3 scarlet
4 light green

Group B
1 pinkish-violet
2 lilac
3 dusky pink
4 white

Group E
1 pinkish-violet
2 dusky blue
3 violet
4 bluish-grey

Group D
1 shocking pink
2 dusky pink
3 yellow
4 bright blue
5 orange
6 lime green
7 light grey

Group C
1 black
2 white

Colour-rosette test

words, it should be an emotional response rather than an intellectual decision based on conditioning or 'good taste'.

Each coloured rosette corresponds to a particular family of fragrances and its corresponding 'personality tendency':

Extrovert mood tendency — fresh or green scents (orange/yellow/scarlet/light green) *Group A*

Introvert mood tendency — oriental notes (pinkish-violet/lilac/dusky pink/white) *Group B*

Emotionally ambivalent mood tendency (highly changeable) — floral-dry fragrances (black/white) *Group C*

Emotionally ambivalent, emphasizing extrovert mood tendency − floral-fruity notes (shocking pink/dusky pink/yellow/bright blue/orange/lime green/light grey) *Group D*

Emotionally ambivalent, emphasizing introverted mood tendency − oriental-floral scents (pinkish-violet/dusky blue/violet/bluish-grey) *Group E*

Emotionally stable with extroverted mood tendency − chypre notes which are reminiscent of damp woods after rain, usually with a fruity or floral tinge (shocking pink/dark red/deep pink/amber/turquoise) *Group F*

Emotionally stable with introverted mood tendency − scents with synthetic aldehydic notes and floral undertones (deep blue/yellow/white) *Group G*

There is one other rosette where the colours are a harmonious blend of yellow ochre, olive green and terracotta. This combination is reminiscent of the current mood of the times − the search for a new connection with Mother Earth. From my own experience, those who choose the earthy rosette are particularly drawn to ethnic fragrances with a predominance of patchouli, vetiver, cedarwood or perhaps frankincense. This choice often indicates that the individual is receptive to the aromas of organic essences in general.

Should a person prefer two or even three rosettes, this indicates that the perfume user may find something that appeals to them in two or more families of scent. As a psychological guide to individual perfume preference, the colour rosette test is thought to be at least 80 per cent accurate. Additionally, it can be predicted with 90 per cent accuracy which fragrances will be rejected. In this way, two or three appropriate fragrance samples can be offered to the customer − an approach which guards against the problem of odour fatigue, which can result in a disastrous (and expensive) perfumery purchase.

Aromatherapy massage blends

The art of aromatherapy has been extensively written about elsewhere (see the Suggested Reading list in the appendix). However, it seems appropriate to include basic instructions for preparing your own massage oil blends which can be rubbed all over the body after a bath or shower (warmth and moisture facilitate the penetration of oils), or they can be used as a facial treatment. Plant essences diluted in the finest quality vegetable oils (for example, almond, sunflower, safflower, apricot kernel) make wonderful skin-care agents. However, unless you are already well versed in aromatherapy, it is best to use only the plant essences recommended below for facial skin-care. Certain essential oils and absolutes used in high concentration may irritate the softer, more sensitive skin of the face. Choose from the following:

Chamomile – all skin types, but use in the lowest concentration.

Frankincense – for oily skin, it helps to balance secretion of sebum.

Lavender – suits all skin types.

Neroli – all skin types.

Rose otto – all skin types. If blended 50/50 with frankincense it makes a good rejuvenating mixture for mature skin.

Sandalwood – especially helpful for dry skin.

Most other essences can be blended into body massage oils, but do check the aromatic repertory for any contra-indications (see Chapter 3).

Recommended dilutions

Body oils – to each teaspoonful (approximately 5 ml) of

vegetable base oil, add between 1 and 3 drops of essential oil, depending on the odour intensity of the essence.

Facial oils — to each teaspoonful (5 ml) of base oil, add 1 drop of essential oil. You may find that 1 drop per 2 teaspoons (10 ml) of base oil is sufficient for the stronger smelling essences of rose, neroli and chamomile. When using these essences in blends, as little as 1 drop per 25 ml of vegetable oil may be sufficient.

Refer to the odour intensity guide on page 81.

Aromatic baths

Essential oils can also be used in the bath to aid relaxation or to ease muscular aches and pains (refer to the therapeutic information in Chapter 3). Any of the oil- or alcohol-based perfume blends suggested in Chapter 6 can be used in the bath if desired. Alternatively, use neat essential oils. Add between 4 and 8 drops (depending on the strength of the aroma) to the bath after it has been drawn; agitate the water to aid dispersal. If you add the essential oil whilst the water is running, the aromatic molecules will evaporate before you enter the bath.

If you have dry skin, you may also wish to add a few teaspoons of vegetable oil to the water; although this will float on the surface, you can massage the vegetable oil into your skin whilst sitting in the bath. A light film will remain on the skin even after drying with a towel, unless you dry yourself too vigorously.

Odour intensity guide

The following essences have powerful aromas and dominate blends unless used in small quantities. The amount suggested for each essence is per 10 ml of jojoba oil, light coconut oil or alcohol for perfume strength blends, per 15 ml of vegetable oil for massage blends and per 100 ml of water for room perfumes, aftershave mixtures or colognes. Where alcohol is available for making colognes, the quantity of essential oil is the same as for water.

Angelica: 1 or 2 drops

Basil: (room scent only) 1 or 2 drops

Black pepper: 1 or 2 drops

Cardamom: 1 drop

Chamomile: 1 or 2 drops

Cinnamon bark (*room perfume only*): 2 or 3 drops

Clove (*room perfume only*): 2 or 3 drops

Elemi: 1 or 2 drops

Eucalyptus: 1 drop

Fennel: 1 or 2 drops

Frankincense: 1 to 3 drops

Galbanum: 1 or 2 drops

Ginger: 1 drop

Jasmine: 1 or 2 drops

Lemongrass: 1 drop

Myrrh: 1 or 2 drops

Neroli: 2 to 4 drops

Orange flower absolute: 1 or 2 drops

Peppermint: 1 or 2 drops

Rose absolute: 2 to 4 drops

Rose otto: 1 to 3 drops

Tagetes: less than one drop (extremely difficult to work with)

You may also find the following aromatics overpowering unless carefully balanced out with other essences according

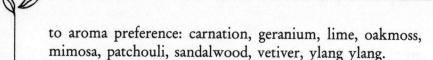

to aroma preference: carnation, geranium, lime, oakmoss, mimosa, patchouli, sandalwood, vetiver, ylang ylang.

Room scents

You will find that blending environmental fragrances is easier than blending skin perfumes because exact quantities are not crucial. Moreover, your blends will always smell 'true', they will not be altered by your own body scent. You will also be able to enjoy blends containing stimulating spices such as clove and cinnamon bark, essences which are too strong to be used on the skin. You could also try a predominantly minty blend – although refreshing, hardly suitable as a skin perfume, unless you delight in smelling like a Polo mint! Whatever your inclination, it is a good idea to start with making room scents (see Chapter 7), thus familiarizing yourself with different essential oils and their aroma effects, and to progress from there to perfumes if you wish. After all, not everyone likes to wear perfume, but a great many people do appreciate a subtly fragrant room.

Aroma-test your blends

Before mixing a quantity of skin or room perfume as directed in the following two chapters, you need to find out whether or not the blend is compatible with your personality or present mood. There is nothing more disappointing than discovering that an enchanting-sounding blend is totally out of synch with your own expectations, especially if you are left with a full bottle of the offending brew. No doubt you will also wish to experiment with blends of your own devising. Here, then, are a few economical methods for smell-testing your aromatic concoctions.

1 Put a drop or two of each essential oil on a damp cotton wool bud, a smelling paper or a piece of blotting paper. Before smelling, waft the sample around for a moment to encourage vaporization of the essences. If you dislike the effect, you have wasted only a small amount of essential oil.

2 A more accurate guide would be to mix the sample combination of oils (up to 6 drops in total) in a teaspoon of light coconut oil or jojoba and apply to the inside of your wrist before smelling. The oils then have the chance to interact with your skin chemistry. If you like the effect, mix to perfume strength.

3 For the testing of aromatic waters and room perfumes, add up to 6 drops of essential oil to 2 teaspoons of warm water and mix well. If you are not very keen on the effect, but don't dislike it too much, sprinkle the mixture over the carpet. It will impart a pleasant aroma without damaging the fabric. However, if the mixture contains a goodly proportion of valerian essence, put it on a tissue and offer it to the cat — she will love it!

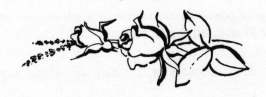

6 Alluring Skin Perfumes

The perfume formulae in this chapter are merely a starting point. Even if you love the fragrance of a particular blend, it must also harmonize with your own natural body scent, so be prepared to play around with the ingredients until you create a perfume that is right for you. You may also find it helpful to refer to the 'blends well with' note at the end of each essential oil profile in Chapter 3. Of course, only the highest quality essences and absolutes should be used. A fine perfume cannot be created from second rate oils.

It is also important to realize that it cannot be guaranteed that your blends will be in perfect accord each time, for no two batches of the same type of essential oil (French lavender, for instance) will smell identical. Like wine, essential oils have good, bad and indifferent years; they are also influenced by temperature, humidity and age. So, although the blends suggested in this book were harmonious at the time of their creation (during the cool, wetter-than-normal Welsh summer of 1993), it may not be possible to reproduce exactly the same resonance with a different batch of essences in a different climate. Aroma chemicals, on the other hand, are more or less stable in this respect. However, once you become familiar with essential oils and confident about blending, I feel sure you will develop the ability to adjust the quantities according to the odour nuance of your particular materials. Indeed, as you will discover, although there is a technique to the art of creating perfumes, intuition or instinct play a greater part.

The families of scent

Most perfumes can be categorized according to their essential character: floral, chypre, green, oriental, or leather (though most will have overtones of another as well). The first four families of scent can be produced entirely from plant essences. However, the leather-like perfumes almost always contain synthetic chemicals or animal extracts. We shall therefore ignore these and concentrate on the others, which offer a vast range of possibilities.

Floral – either a single floral note such as rose or carnation, or a harmonious bouquet without any particular flower predominating. Essentially feminine.

Chypre – a dark green blend, often with a floral and/or citrus tinge; reminiscent of woods after rain. The chypres are long-lasting and sensuous and can appeal to both men and women.

Green – fresh and clear, reminiscent of the great outdoors. The greens may be largely composed of evergreen essences such as cedarwood and juniper, or galbanum, heightened by clary sage or lavender and perhaps a breeze of lime. Eau de cologne blends, composed almost entirely of citrus essences, also fall into this category (though 'fresh' would be a better description). A cooling and enlivening group of fragrances, popular with men, and essentially androgynous.

Oriental – A tenacious, overtly seductive blend composed of deeply resonating esences of woods and resins, exotic florals and spices, and of luscious fruits. A style of perfume which can be adapted to suit either sex. Strictly for the bold at heart!

Basic procedure for perfume-making

Many of the perfume blends suggested in the aromatic formulae section beginning on page 88 do not contain a base or a top note as such, though usually they will include a bridging essence, one which resonates slightly above or below the middle or base range, e.g. ylang ylang (middle to base), clary sage (middle to top). Refer to pages 69–70.

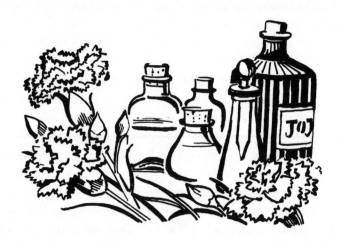

Oil-based perfume

Fill a 10 ml dark glass bottle almost to the top with jojoba or light coconut oil. Build your perfume slowly drop by drop, shaking the bottle well after each addition and smelling as you go. You will need 15-20 drops of essential oil altogether. Begin with the base note (if included), then develop the heart of the perfume and finally the top note.

Once mixed, your perfume needs to be left for one or two weeks to mature. Keep in a cool dark place, but remember to shake the bottle once a day to facilitate the process. At the end of the maturation period, the blend will have lost its 'raw' overtones and will smell much more rounded.

Alcohol-based perfume

Fill a 10 ml dark glass bottle almost to the top with ethanol and proceed as for oil-based perfume.

You can add a little distilled water to alcohol-based blends if you wish to make the alcohol go farther. Indeed, all commercial perfumes contain a small percentage of water. However, it can be a tricky operation; add too much (or the right amount too quickly) and your perfume will become irretrievably cloudy. Generally speaking, you can add up to 5 drops of water to every 5 ml of alcohol/essential oil mix. The most important thing is to add the water *after* the essential oil has fully dissolved in the alcohol. Add one drop of water at a time (use a pipette) and shake well after each addition.

Hair perfume

Generally speaking, unless a natural perfume contains a good proportion of a highly tenacious oil such as jasmine, sandalwood or carnation, it will not have the staying power of a high-class commercial product which may contain a powerful chemical fixative.

As well as applying perfume to your skin, you could therefore apply it to the ends of your hair (if you have enough hair, that is!) for extra scent. Hair is a marvellous fixative for perfume; it also intensifies the fragrance. The light citrus or green scents are especially enhanced by the subtle odour of hair. Try to avoid getting any perfume on the scalp as the skin is sensitive there.

Unless your hair is thick and heavy, an oil-based perfume may leave a greasy feel. For this reason, an alcohol-based product (or an aromatic water — see page 97) may be the best choice. Alternatively, you could use neat essential oils. The essences will not damage your hair, nor will they leave a greasy film. A few neat essences could be blended together in a bottle to make a complex perfume, or you could use a favourite single essence such as rose, jasmine, sandalwood or ylang ylang.

If you are a man with a goodly growth of beard, then you could perfume your whiskers! To my mind, there is something enticing about a well groomed, subtly fragrant beard.

Aromatic formulae

Most of the blends in this section will appeal to people of either sex (except, perhaps, some of the florals which are essentially feminine). Generally speaking, however, the woods, spices, citrus or resins should be emphasized in 'masculine' blends rather than the flowers, although the floral essences can form an interesting background note, especially lavender and geranium which impart a refreshing, uplifting quality. In the love potions section on page 94, however, I have separated out the masculine from the feminine blends, though do feel free to wear a perfume which is meant for the opposite sex if it appeals to you. In this book, rules are meant to be broken!

IMPORTANT: Quantities for all the following blends are given in drops per 10 ml of oil or alcohol.

Flowers of Eden (Floral)

The following essences and absolutes may appeal to you just as they are: rose absolute, rose otto, orange flower absolute, carnation, jasmine, ylang ylang. Any of these heavy florals can be lifted by blending with equal quantities of lavender or bergamot, or a little of each according to preference. Or try any of the following blends:

1 Jasmine 3, clary sage 6, lavender 6.

2 Ylang Ylang 2, sandalwood 10, lavender 5, coriander 3.

3 Rose absolute 4, neroli 4, bergamot 5, mandarin 4.

4 Jasmine 3, ylang ylang 6, geranium (or lavender) 6.

5 Ylang ylang 8, orange flower absolute 2 (or neroli 4), geranium 5.

6 Carnation 4, lavender 6, grapefruit 5.

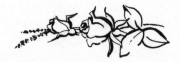

From the Wildwood (Chypre)

The following essences may appeal to you just as they are: cedarwood, sandalwood, patchouli. You might like to lift the fragrance a little by adding up to 5 drops of clary sage or lavender to 15 drops of any of the aforementioned oils. Otherwise, try one or two of the following complex blends:

1 Cedarwood 8, vetiver 4, clary sage 4, rose otto 1, petitgrain 3.

2 Sandalwood 6, vetiver 3, patchouli 2, carnation 3, bergamot 6.

3 Frankincense 6, oakmoss 3, elemi 2, lavender 6.

4 Cypress 2, clary sage 2, geranium 3, sandalwood 8.

5 Oakmoss 3, rose absolute 10.

6 Sandalwood 5, oakmoss 3, mimosa 6, lavender 6.

Of the Glade (Green)

An equal quantity of lavender and bergamot makes a refreshing fragrance, or try some of the following blends:

1 Oakmoss 2, patchouli 1, lavender 10, bergamot 7.

2 Juniper 8, galbanum 1, clary sage 4, lavender 6.

3 Juniper 8, clary sage 4, bergamot 8.

4 Oakmoss 3, galbanum 1, lavender 6, neroli 3, lemon 4, lime 2.

5 Cedarwood 5, juniper 5, mimosa 4, lavender 6.

6 Vetiver 4, clary sage 10, orange flower absolute 2 (or neroli 4).

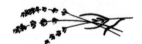

Dreams of Mandalay (Oriental)

An equal quantity of ylang ylang and mandarin makes an exotic fragrance. Or why not be bolder still and try one or two of the following head-spinners:

1 Ylang ylang 7, black pepper 3, mandarin 5.

2 Frankincense 5, elemi 1, geranium 3, bergamot 6, mandarin 6.

3 Ylang ylang 5, rose otto 2, orange 4, coriander 8.

4 Frankincense 3, jasmine 3, bergamot 6, black pepper 3.

5 Carnation 3, coriander 6, mandarin 6.

6 Sandalwood 9, rose absolute 6, ginger 1, orange 4.

Essential oil concentrates

For a more interesting, multi-faceted perfume, you could add several drops of an essential oil concentrate (a mixture of undiluted essences) to your aromatic concoctions. A few of the concentrates suggested below mimic some of the more expensive (or elusive) absolutes to a degree and can therefore be used in their place. For instance, there is a mock oakmoss and a mock carnation blend. Although you could mix neat essential oils together in one bottle to make a concentrate, this can be a fairly costly exercise. Therefore, the best alternative method is to dilute the oils at the rate of 50 drops of essential oil to 5 ml (approximately 100 drops) of oil or alcohol.

As a rough guide, 4 drops of concentrate are equal to approximately 1 drop of undiluted essential oil.

Included in each section are two perfume strength blends which incorporate the concentrate. You will notice that a few of the blends are diluted in home-made vanilla oil rather than plain jojoba, light coconut oil or alcohol. Vanilla absolute is extremely costly as well as being difficult to obtain. However, the infused oil works almost as well, and at a fraction of the cost (see the recipe on page 94).

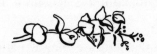

Wood concentrates

1 Sandalwood 30, vetiver 15, patchouli 6.

2 Cedarwood 33, vetiver 12, patchouli 5.

Suggested perfumes

1 10 ml infused vanilla oil as a base (or use plain jojoba, light coconut oil or alcohol), 40 drops of wood concentrate No. 1, rose absolute 4 (or 2 drops rose otto), lavender 2, bergamot 3.

2 40 drops wood concentrate No. 2, mimosa 3, clary sage 5.

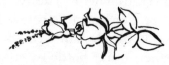

Mock oakmoss concentrates

1 Cedarwood 20, vetiver 10, clary sage 8, petitgrain 12.

2 Cedarwood 20, vetiver 10, patchouli 5, clary sage 15.

Suggested perfumes

1 40 drops mock oakmoss concentrate No. 1 or No. 2, neroli 4 (or 2 drops orange flower absolute), lavender 2, bergamot 2, lemon 2.

2 40 drops mock oakmoss concentrate No. 1 or No. 2, lavender 4, geranium 3, ylang ylang 3.

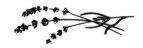

Green concentrates

1 Lavender 30, bergamot 10, oakmoss 10.

2 Lavender 30, galbanum 10, bergamot 10.

Suggested perfumes

1 40 drops green concentrate No. 1, petitgrain 4, lemon 4, lime 2.

2 40 drops green concentrate No. 2, jasmine 3, geranium 2, grapefruit 5.

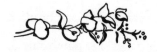

Citrus concentrates

1 Bergamot 30, lemon 12, neroli 6.

2 Bergamot 30, lemon 8, mandarin 6, petitgrain 6.

Suggested perfumes

1 10 ml infused vanilla oil as a base, 50 drops citrus concentrate No. 1, rose absolute 4, ginger 1.

2 40 drops citrus concentrate No. 2, rosemary 5, lavender 5.

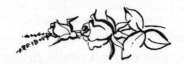

Resin concentrates

1 Frankincense 30, elemi 5, lavender 15.

2 Frankincense 30, myrrh 10, lemon 10.

Suggested perfumes

1 40 drops resin concentrate No. 1, geranium 5, ylang ylang 5.

2 40 drops resin concentrate No. 2, mandarin 5, coriander 5.

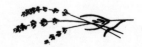

Mock carnation concentrates

1 5 ml infused vanilla oil as a base, ylang ylang 20, black pepper 30.

2 5 ml infused vanilla oil as a base, ylang ylang 15, rose absolute 5, black pepper 30.

3 Ylang ylang 20, black pepper 30.

4 Ylang ylang 15, rose absolute 5, black pepper 30.

Suggested perfumes

1 10 ml infused vanilla oil as a base, 40 drops of mock carnation concentrate No. 1 or 2, angelica 3, mandarin 5.

2 40 drops mock carnation concentrate No. 3 or 4, geranium 3, grapefruit 2, lemon 5.

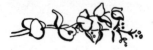

Infused oil of vanilla

This is the base oil mentioned in some of the previous blends and can be used with any vanilla-compatible blends.

You will need 50 ml light coconut oil or jojoba, a vanilla pod and a clear glass jar with a tight fitting lid. The method is simple: cut the vanilla pod into small pieces and place in the jar. Cover with the oil, seal tightly and leave outside in the sun or on a warm radiator or boiler for about six weeks, bringing the jar indoors at night. Give the jar a good shake every time you pass by to facilitate the infusion process. When the oil smells fragrant, strain through muslin and store in a dark glass bottle. The oil will keep for at least one year.

Love potions

The following blends will work wonders if combined with an attractive partner and one other essential ingredient – imagination!

Potions for women to use

1 10 ml infused vanilla oil as a base, ylang ylang 8, rose absolute 4, lime 3.

2 Carnation 4, coriander 6, bergamot 6.

3 Sandalwood 6, angelica 2, clary sage 7.

4 Neroli 4, jasmine 3, lavender 3, mandarin 5.

5 Jasmine 4, clary sage 5, bergamot 8.

6 Sandalwood 10, rose absolute 5.

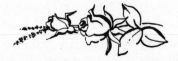

Potions for men to use

1 Cedarwood 10, rosemary 5, orange 5.

2 Sandalwood 10, angelica 2, coriander 5.

3 Rose absolute 4 (or rose otto 2), ginger 3, coriander 12.

4 Jasmine 4, patchouli 7, black pepper 4.

5 Carnation 4, frankincense 9, cardamom 1.

6 Vetiver 4, cedarwood 8, jasmine 3.

7 Oakmoss 3, sandalwood 10, rose otto 2 (or rose absolute 4).

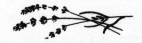

Solid perfumes

You may prefer to make solid perfumes which are easier to carry around whilst travelling. They are very simple to make. You will need:

25–30 drops essential oil
2 teaspoonsful (10 ml) jojoba or light coconut oil
1 rounded teaspoonful grated beeswax

Blend the essential oils with the jojoba or coconut oil as on page 86. Melt the beeswax in a small heatproof bowl placed over a saucepan of simmering water. Remove from the heat and stir in the perfume blend. Pour into a small sterilized glass pot (it will set firm within a minute or two), cover tightly and label with the perfume and date. (When sterilizing it is best to use the 'boiling' method as sterilizing tablets can leave a faint odour of chlorine. Place the little glass pots in a saucepan of cold water, cover and bring to the boil. Turn down the heat and simmer for ten minutes. Remove from the heat but leave tightly covered until you can lift out the pots without burning your fingers. Shake out as much water as possible then dry with a spotlessly clean tea towel immediately before pouring in the wax perfume. The perfume will keep for at least six months if kept in a cool dark place.

The honey-scented beeswax adds its own subtle fragrance to the blend. If the blend is vanilla-compatible, you could use infused vanilla oil with the beeswax instead of plain oil. Any of the previously mentioned blends can be incorporated into the beeswax base, but you will need to adjust the quantity of essential oil accordingly, to bring it to a total of 25–30 drops. Of course, you may prefer the fragrance of a single essence. My own favourites are jasmine, rose otto, carnation and sandalwood which are lovely as loners, but can be enhanced by vanilla.

How to apply perfume

Perfume is usually applied to the pulse points – behind the ears, the sides of the neck, the inside of the wrists, the elbow creases, behind the knees and around the ankles – as these points help to radiate the fragrance. There are those who swear that perfume actually smells better when applied to these special places. However, don't overdo it, especially when using the come-hither florientals. Fragrance should whisper, not shout!

Aromatic waters

Even though essential oils are thought to be insoluble in water, I prefer to regard them as *partially* water-soluble. Rosewater and orange flower water, for example, are produced as a result of water taking up the essential oil's fragrance during the distillation process. Similarly, highly acceptable aromatic waters (made to cologne strength — 100 drops of essential oil to 100 ml water) can be made by mixing together essential oils and water. However, the mixture will need to be poured through a coffee filter paper because most of the essential oil will float on the surface. If you prefer not to filter your aromatic waters (after all, a lot of oil gets left behind on the filter paper), then you will need to shake the bottle each time before use to disperse the essential oil. Alternatively, if you can obtain perfume grade alcohol, use this as a base for your colognes. In this instance there is no need to filter the mixture as the oils are entirely soluble in alcohol. Aromatic waters will keep for about three months.

Any of the spicy aromatic decoctions suggested in Chapter 7 can also be used as a base for a cologne. As mentioned on page xv some of the spice oils, cinnamon and clove in particular, are too harsh for the skin. However, aromatic decoctions of the same spices can be safely used as a splash-on product, but it may be wise to carry out a patch test first (see page xiii).

Making water-based blends

Fill a 100 ml dark glass bottle with distilled water, orange flower water, rosewater, an aromatic decoction, or a 50/50 mixture of any two. Build the fragrance gradually by adding a few drops of essential oil at a time, shaking the bottle and smelling as you go. Add up to 100 drops of essential oil in all (the average strength for most colognes). Allow the mixture to ripen for one or two weeks before use. Keep in a cool dark place, but remember to shake well each day to facilitate the infusion process. When ready, pour through a damp coffee filter paper (a dry filter paper will absorb too much of the liquid), rebottle and label with the blend and date.

Making alcohol-based blends

Pour 80 ml ethanol through a funnel into a dark glass bottle. Add a few drops of essential oil at a time, shaking the bottle and smelling as you go, adding up to 100 drops in all. Then add 20 ml distilled water, a few drops at a time, shaking well after each addition. If you add the water too quickly, the blend will become irretrievably cloudy. Allow the mixture to ripen for one or two weeks, remembering to shake the bottle daily. At the end of this period the cologne is ready to use.

Suggested blends

Except for those blends which are based on rosewater, orange flower water or an aromatic decoction, many of the following colognes can be made with distilled water or alcohol.

1 Lavender 50, bergamot 50.

2 Rosemary 25, bergamot 25, lemon 50.

3 Patchouli 30, ylang ylang 40, geranium 20.

4 Lavender 30, clary sage 30, bergamot 30, rose absolute 10.

5 Ginger 5, coriander 30, bergamot 30, lemon 30, lime 5.

6 100 ml clove or cinnamon decoction, 30 drops coriander, 30 drops mandarin.

7 100 ml vanilla decoction, rose absolute 10, ylang ylang 10, bergamot 20.

8 50 ml orange flower water, 50 ml rosewater, geranium 25, orange 50.

9 Rosemary 15, lavender 30, orange 30, lemon 20.

10 Rosemary 30, clary sage 20, lavender 40, peppermint 5.

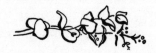

Eau de Cologne blends

1 Elemi 3, bergamot 30, geranium 5, orange 25, coriander 10, petitgrain 10, lavender 10, lime 5.

2 Rose absolute 10, neroli 10, grapefruit 10, lemon 10, orange 10, mandarin 10, lavender 10, bergamot 25.

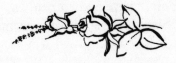

How to apply aromatic waters

These can be used in the same way as commercial products – splashed on after a bath or shower, brushed through the hair or sprinkled over clothes. However, the best way to apply an aromatic water is to spray it on, using an atomizer which can be purchased from a good chemist or the perfume counter of a department store.

Aftershave

Some men are apprehensive about smelling of anything other than medicated soap, though perhaps they could be tempted by a gently antiseptic, yet pleasantly aromatic aftershave formula. Commercial products usually contain a high concentration of alcohol (and synthetic fragrance) which can irritate the sensitive skin of the face. Therefore, the simple aftershave mixtures suggested here are alcohol-free. They contain a small quantity of cider vinegar which helps to restore the skin's natural acid/alkali balance.

Not all essential oils are suitable for aftershave blends as many are too strong for facial skin, especially some of the spices. So choose between one and three oils from the following: cedarwood, chamomile, coriander, cypress, frankincense, geranium, juniper, lavender, marjoram, neroli, palmarosa, patchouli, rose, rosemary, sandalwood, vetiver, ylang ylang.

Blending aftershave

Pour 300 ml rosewater, orange flower water or distilled water into a dark glass bottle. Add 1 or 2 teaspoons of cider vinegar and shake well. Then add between 3 and 5 drops of essential oil. The aftershave is then ready to use. There is no need to filter the blend as long as you remember to shake the bottle each time before use.

Suggested aftershave blends

1 Frankincense 3, coriander 2.

2 Sandalwood 3, palmarosa 1.

3 Patchouli 2, lavender 3.

4 Rosemary 2, marjoram 1, cedarwood 2.

5 Vetiver 2, sandalwood 2, lavender 1.

6 Vetiver 1, cypress 1, juniper 2.

7 Chamomile 1, geranium 1, lavender 2.

8 Frankincense 3, ylang ylang 2.

9 Frankincense 3, rose 2.

10 Cedarwood 2, neroli 1.

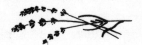

Perfume gifts

When giving perfume, an aromatic water or aftershave as a gift, it is vital to ascertain the person's perfume preference, which means you will need to know them extremely well. If in doubt, give them something else, or take a chance and opt for fresh high notes in an aqueous or alcohol-base rather than a heavy, clinging oil-based brew. For instance, go for a traditional eau de cologne blend as most people find this harmony agreeable. Similarly, when mixing a room fragrance (see Chapter 7) for someone you do not know well, opt for a simple duet or trio composed of citrus or green notes rather than a deeply resonating earthy or floriental extravaganza.

It's all in the name

Well, not quite, but an imaginative name adds to the enchantment of an aromatic concoction, especially when presented as a gift. Sometimes I think of the name first, then try to create an evocative fragrance to suit. At other times, a new blend speaks for itself. Here, then, are some of my own ideas just to get you started. No doubt you will be inspired in many other directions. Have fun!

Enchanted Summer	Lady Chatterley	Lionheart
		Firebird
Dreams of Amethyst	Truly, Madly, Deeply	Dryad
Whispering Sands	Titania	Harlequin
	Tamlin	Bedouin
Green on Green	Moments	Mosaic
Forever Jade	Timeless	Kaleidoscope
	Moonchild	Jabberwocky

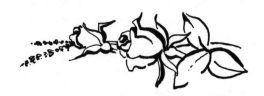

7 Mood-Enhancing Room Scents

Although there are a number of methods for perfuming rooms, to my mind, the traditional essential oil vaporizer or 'burner' is the most beautiful. 'Burner', however, is a misnomer because essential oils should never be overheated as this causes the aromatic vapour to evaporate far too quickly. A well-designed vaporizer will warm the oil just enough to enable the aroma to gradually waft around the room.

While most essential oil vaporizers are earthenware, there are a few glass, porcelain or marble versions on the market. Most vaporizers resemble small pots with decorative shapes cut out of the sides of allow a free flow of air around the nightlight candle placed inside. A small, sometimes detachable, reservoir fits over the nightlight and is filled with water with a few drops of essential oil floated on the surface. The gentle heat of the candle releases the aromatic vapour. Alternatively, a few drops of essential oil can be added to a radiator humidifier, but the odour effect may be weaker than that obtained by using a purpose-designed vaporizer.

There is a high-tech alternative to the humble nightlight vaporizer in the shape of the electric fragrancer. Here, a few drops of undiluted essential oil are dropped on to a ceramic or filter surface which is kept at a constant warm

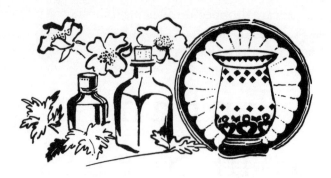

temperature. These gadgets are particularly suitable for the workplace and certainly much safer than nightlights for children's bedrooms. The drawback is that many electric fragrancers are designed to take only neat essential oil, which means you have to forgo the delights of vaporizing the aromatic waters and spicy decoctions suggested in the recipe section.

The most recent innovation is the stream diffuser. A cold-air pump blows minute droplets of neat essential oil into the atmosphere. Although manufacturers extol the virtues of this method on the grounds that heat radically alters the chemical structure of essential oils, I am not convinced that it is a superior method. Indeed, *gentle* heat actually enhances the aroma of essential oils and other aromatic materials. Stream diffusers are often exorbitantly priced, which says it all.

Light bulb perfumery

It is said that women of questionable repute perfume their light bulbs with patchouli oil! However, no longer need you be engaged in the oldest profession to explore the joys of light bulb perfumery, for it has become quite a respectable practice. You may be able to obtain a fragrance ring which is a ceramic disc that balances over the top of the light bulb.

The essences are dropped on the ring and the warmth from the bulb releases the aromatic vapour. Alternatively, simply rub a few drops of essence on to a *cold* light bulb (a desk lamp works well), then turn on the light.

Scented candles

Although it is possible to buy scented candles, few contain natural essential oils. Even when genuine essential oil candles are available, the choice is usually limited to a handful of aromas: lavender, ylang ylang, sandalwood and perhaps one or two other popular scents. While candle-making kits are available from some craft shops, it is much easier, and a great deal cheaper, to buy one very fat candle and a few of your favourite essential oils. The method is simple. First light the candle, wait a few moments for the wax on the top edge of the candle to melt, then blow it out and immediately add a few drops of essential oil to the molten wax (the fatter the candle, the bigger the pool of wax) before re-lighting.

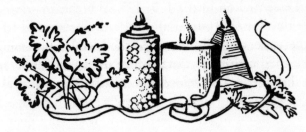

IMPORTANT: Essential oil is highly flammable, so if you attempt to add this whilst the candle is still burning, it will flare up, leaving in its wake a puff of black smoke.

It is also important to keep the wick trimmed very short, otherwise the flame will be too big and the aromatic vapour relatively short-lived. If the pool of wax is big enough and the flame low enough, the aroma will continue to diffuse for at least an hour. Once all the oil has evaporated, you may wish to ring the changes by adding a different essence or a blend of two of three (extinguishing the flame first).

Blending for the vaporizer

Should you have chosen the type of electric vaporizer which cannot take oils suspended in water, you will need to use 3 or 4 drops of neat essential oil, which should be enough to perfume a room of up to 3 metres square. For a much larger space, you may need up to 15 drops. For complex blends of more than two or three essences, it may be easier to make a concentrate by mixing several oils together, using just a few drops of the blend on the ceramic or filter surface. If you use more than 6 drops of essential oil, the aroma can be over-powering in a small room. However, before blending the oils, it is important to ensure that the effect will be pleasing, otherwise you may have wasted a large amount of essential oil, so it would be wise to aroma test your blends (see page 82).

To make blends for the nightlight vaporizer; mix 15–20 drops of essential oil into a 100–125 ml bottle of water (tap water is fine for this purpose). Shake the bottle and fill the oil burner reservoir with some of the blend. Do remember to shake the bottle each time before use to aid dispersal of the oil. For special occasions, try mixing the essential oils with rosewater or orange flower water, which is especially lovely with floral or citrus essences or with tiny quantities of spice oils. Alternatively, vaporize an aromatic decoction (prepared from whole spices), with the addition of essential oils if desired (see page 120).

Aromatherapeutic blending

You may be happy with fun blends most of the time, perhaps based on the four families of scent described in the previous chapter. However, there may be times when you feel in need of something more, a personalized blend of aromatics to balance your physical and emotional state. If you have a bedroom to yourself, you could permeate the room with the fragrance before you go to sleep (the best time for aromatherapy), or have the vaporizer in the bathroom whilst you luxuriate in a warm bath, or simply vaporize the oils in the room where you happen to be working or relaxing.

The aromatherapeutic blends suggested here are based on the principles of Ayurveda, the traditional medicine of India which is believed to be at least 5,000 years old. Aromatic oils have always played a part in this comprehensive system of bodymind healing which encompasses diet, herbs, massage, yoga, meditation and much more besides. Should you wish to delve more deeply into Ayurveda, I suggest you obtain a copy of Dr Deepak Chopra's excellent book entitled *Perfect Health, The Complete Mind/Body Guide*.

The principles of Ayurveda

According to Ayurveda, the human bodymind is influenced by five basic principles which equate to the elements of air, fire, water and earth with the fifth principle known as ether or 'space'. This could also be described as the spiritual aspect of our being, or simply 'vibration'. By mixing different pairs of elements, we arrive at the three *doshas* or major operating principles. The three doshas are called Vata (ether and air), Pitta (fire and water) and Kapha (earth and water). Although the doshas regulate thousands of processes in the bodymind complex, they have three basic functions:

Vata – controls movement, i.e. respiration, blood circulation, digestion and the central nervous system.

Pitta – controls metabolism, i.e. the way we process food, air and water throughout the entire system.

Kapha – controls structure, i.e. the formation of muscle, fat, bone, and sinew.

The three doshas are interrelated; when one dosha becomes unbalanced, all three begin to move out of balance to some degree, depending on our individual constitution. Generally speaking, however, by observing our symptoms and state of mind, we can identify which dosha is most troubled and choose the appropriate blend of aromatics to help bring us back into balance. Of course, serious imbalances will need to be investigated by a qualified health practitioner as diet and other factors will need to be taken into account.

Most people lean towards one particular dosha. For instance, there is the so-called Vata type who is generally fast moving, quick thinking and nervy; the fiery Pitta type tends to blow hot and cold; whereas the Kapha type is usually calm and down-to-earth. Of course, few people are totally true to type, with most of us displaying a mixture of two predominant doshas. There is also the rare individual who expresses with equal intensity all three doshas – wonderful if they are in balance, but extremely difficult for the person (and those around) if they are not!

An individual can also move into any one of the dosha states to a greater or less degree, irrespective of 'type'. Following an operation, for instance, even the fiery Pitta and airy Vata can become lethargic (an excess of Kapha) during the recovery period. Conversely, the stolid Kapha can become angry and aggressive (an excess of Pitta) in extreme circumstances. Here, then, are both the positive and the negative bodymind states associated with each of the doshas:

Balanced Vata state – imaginative, sensitive, spontaneous, resilient, exhilarated.

Unbalanced Vata state – nervous tension, mood swings, scattered thoughts, insomnia, disturbed sleep, anxiety, depression, PMS, short attention span, loss of mental focus, impatience, sensitivity to noise, muscular pain, constipation, high blood pressure, low stamina, intolerance to cold and windy weather.

Balanced Pitta state – intellectual, confident, enterprising, joyous.

Unbalanced Pitta state – anger, hostility, violent outbursts, self-criticism, resentment, argumentative, tyrannical behaviour, intolerance of delays, excessive hunger or thirst, hot flushes (during menopause), fiery pre-menstrual distress, heartburn, ulcers, sour body odours, intolerance to humid summer weather or the electric atmosphere before a storm.

Balanced Kapha state – calm, easy-going, courageous, forgiving, loving.

Unbalanced Kapha state – mental inertia, lethargy, possessiveness, stupor, depression, procrastination, inability to accept change, seasonal affective disorder (winter depression), pre-menstrual lassitude, menstrual fatigue, oversleeping, slow movements, catarrhal, fluid retention, aching joints, heaviness in limbs, frequent colds, intolerance to cold and damp.

Bodymind aromas

Aromas and tastes can be used to help balance the doshas. Indeed, any of the spices and herbs listed below can be used in their dry form and added to food. Of course, you need not fit any of the aforementioned dosha descriptions *exactly* (heaven forbid!) in order for a particular blend of aromas to be used. With a little common sense, it should be easy to ascertain which category of aromas would best suit your needs at a given time.

Vata aromas

When making blends to balance Vata, use a mixture of warm, sweet and sour aromas. Choose at least one aroma from each category:

Warm — angelica, basil, bergamot, cardamom, cedarwood, cinnamon, clove, fennel, frankincense, ginger, marjoram, patchouli, vetiver.

Sweet — chamomile, clary sage, grapefruit, mandarin, jasmine, lavender, orange, palmarosa, rose, sandalwood, vanilla, ylang ylang.

Sour — lemon, lime.

Vata tastes — salty, sour, oily and sweet. For example: salted pistachio nuts (salt and oil), followed by banana, dates and yoghurt (sour and sweet).

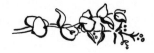

Pitta aromas

When making blends to balance Pitta, use a mixture of sweet and cool aromas. However, you will notice that some of the sweet aromas are also warm, e.g. cinnamon or fennel. It is best to keep these in the background, perhaps emphasizing the obviously cool-smelling aromas of lavender, cypress, clary sage or peppermint. Choose at least one aroma from each category:

Sweet — bergamot, cardamom, chamomile, cinnamon, clary sage, coriander, fennel, geranium, jasmine, neroli, sandalwood, ylang ylang.

Cool — clary sage, cypress, lavender, lemongrass, peppermint, petitgrain, pine.

Pitta tastes — bitter, sweet and astringent. For example: a salad containing vegetables such as celery, cucumber and lettuce (bitter and astringent), followed by date and apple crumble with cream (sweet).

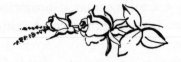

Kapha aromas

When making blends to balance Kapha, use a mixture of warm and spicy aromas. However, many of these oils are also classified as 'sweet', and too much sweet increases Kapha. Therefore it is important to keep the sweeter smelling aromas of bergamot, geranium and coriander, for example, in the background, with greater emphasis placed on the pungent aromas of ginger, black pepper, rosemary and juniper, for example. Choose at least one aroma from each category:

Warm — basil, bergamot, cedarwood, coriander, elemi, frankincense, geranium, marjoram, myrrh, rosemary.

Spicy — black pepper, cardamom, cinnamon, cloves, ginger, juniper.

Kapha tastes — pungent, bitter and astringent. For example: baked potatoes with curried beans (pungent), sprinkled with sesame seeds and served with fenugreek salad sprouts (bitter and astringent).

Getting started

The aromatic concoctions suggested below are based on the simple essential oil and water blends mentioned on page 97.

However, should you prefer to make a concentrate (a mixture of undiluted essences) to be used in an electric fragrancer, simply mix the oils together in approximately the same ratio. For example, where a recipe calls for 4 drops cardamom, 5 drops bergamot, 5 drops ylang ylang and 5 drops lime, simply mix together in a 5 ml or 10 ml bottle equal quantities of the last three oils and a little less cardamom (exact quantities are not at all crucial). Shake well, then use just 3 or 4 drops of the concentrate. Concentrates can also be used in radiator humidifiers, on lightbulbs, in the nightlight vaporizer or to perfume candles (see pages 104–106). Fill the reservoir with water (usually between 20 and 40 ml), then add 4 to 6 drops of concentrate.

Alternatively, instead of blending beforehand, you can simply add several drops from a few bottles of essential oil directly on to the ceramic or filter surface of the electric vaporizer, or directly into the water-filled reservoir of the burner. In this case, you will have to estimate roughly how much of each essence to use when following the recipes outlined below.

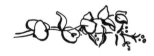

Suggested dosha balancing blends

Quantities for the following blends are given in drops per 100–125 ml water.

Vata

1 Cardamom 4, bergamot 5, ylang ylang 5, lime 5.

2 Frankincense 8, rose 4, cinnamon 3, lemon 5.

3 Vetiver 3, sandalwood 5, bergamot 5, lemon 5.

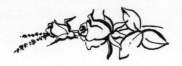

Pitta

1 Ylang ylang 3, clary sage 6, bergamot 4, chamomile 2.

2 Cinnamon 3, neroli 4, lavender 7, geranium 3.

3 Peppermint 3, cypress 6, lavender 9.

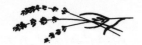

Kapha

1 Basil 8, bergamot 4, rosemary 8.

2 Ginger 4, frankincense 4, coriander 7, marjoram 3.

3 Cedarwood 5, elemi 2, black pepper 5, juniper 5.

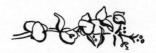

Refining the process of selection

As discussed earlier, most of us display a bodymind state strongly suggestive of more than one dosha. Therefore, Ayurveda combines the three doshas in seven possible ways to arrive at seven other bodymind types (or temporary states of imbalance), which also include the rare three-dosha type — the ratio of Vata, Pitta, and Kapha being nearly even. But with a two-dosha combination, one dosha is usually a little more prominent thus:

Vata/Pitta
Pitta/Vata
Pitta/Kapha
Kapha/Pitta
Vata/Kapha
Kapha/Vata

When choosing aromas to balance two-dosha states, aroma preference and intuition play a major part. As a rough guide, concentrate on the aromas which can be used for either dosha (if possible), but with a little more emphasis on the one which is more prominent.

Suggested two-dosha balancing blends

Vata/Pitta

1 Jasmine 4, lemon 5, bergamot 10.

2 Patchouli 6, lavender 5, geranium 4, lime 4.

Pitta/Vata

1 Ylang ylang 6, clary sage 6, bergamot 6.

2 Chamomile 4, rose 4, lavender 7, lemon 2.

Pitta/Kapha

1 Cinnamon 5, bergamot 9, geranium 4.

2 Lavender 6, rosemary 3, coriander 3, bergamot 6.

Kapha/Pitta

1 Cinnamon 5, coriander 3, geranium 4, bergamot 8.

2 Cardamom 5, lavender 6, bergamot 6, coriander 3.

Vata/Kapha

1 Basil 5, marjoram 5, coriander 8.

2 Frankincense 8, ginger 3, bergamot 8.

Kapha/Vata

1 Cedarwood 5, frankincense 5, juniper 3, bergamot 5.

2 Cedarwood 5, elemi 3, lavender 3, coriander 3, lemon 3.

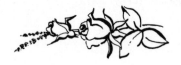

The three-dosha type

Ayurveda offers no clear cut advice to the layperson on balancing all three doshas at the same time. However, it is stressed that when Vata (the 'leader of the doshas') is greatly out of kilter it can mimic Pitta and Kapha. Therefore, if your bodymind state is ambiguous, concentrate on balancing Vata and the other doshas may follow suit. It is said that the true three-dosha type (extremely rare) enjoys lifelong good health, ideal immunity and longevity. But once imbalances start to occur, the individual has a hard task in getting all three doshas back into harmony.

If you are beginning to feel perplexed about the Ayurvedic approach, or would prefer much simpler, less Eastern-smelling mood scents, then read on.

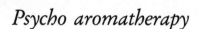

Psycho aromatherapy

Here we concentrate on choosing mood-enhancing essences using the method adopted by most aromatherapists trained in the West. The following at-a-glance reference categorizes a number of essential oils according to their general effect on mood. A single essence or a duet may suit your needs. However, should you also wish to blend according to the top, middle and base note pattern, then refer back to the perfume notes information (pages 69–70). Most importantly, always be guided by your aroma preference. If you dislike the aroma, especially if it evokes a feeling, image or memory you would rather not have, then obviously the effect will be counter productive.

Relaxing

Carnation	Galganum	Neroli
Cedarwood	Juniper	Rose
Chamomile	Mandarin	Sandalwood
Clary sage	Marjoram	Vetiver
Cypress	Myrrh	Ylang ylang

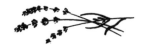

Balancing (stimulates or relaxes according to needs)

Basil	Geranium
Bergamot	Lavender
Frankincense	

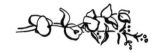

Stimulating

Angelica	Eucalyptus	Palmarosa
Black pepper	Fennel	Peppermint
Cardamom	Ginger	Petitgrain
Cinnamon	Grapefruit	Pine
Cloves	Lime	Rosemary
Elemi	Orange	

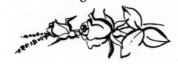

Anti-depressant

Basil	Grapefruit	Orange
Bergamot	Jasmine	Palmarosa
Carnation	Lavender	Patchouli
Chamomile	Lemon	Petitgrain
Clary sage	Lime	Rose
Frankincense	Mandarin	Sandalwood
Geranium	Neroli	Ylang ylang

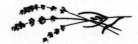

Aphrodisiac

Angelica	Cloves	Patchouli
Cardamom	Coriander	Rose
Carnation	Galbanum	Rosemary
Cedarwood	Ginger	Sandalwood
Cinnamon	Jasmine	Vetiver
Clary sage	Neroli	Ylang ylang

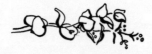

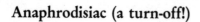

Anaphrodisiac (a turn-off!)

Camphor   Marjoram

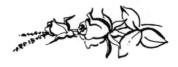

Mental stimulant
(for clarity of thought)

Basil   Peppermint
Cardamom   Pine
Coriander   Rosemary
Eucalyptus

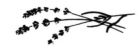

Suggested blends

The following blends are composed of only two or three essences. Therefore, the drops can be added directly to the water-filled vaporizer, used neat in the electric fragrancer, or added to the molten wax of a candle (see page 105). Should you prefer to make up a larger quantity of room scent to be used in the nightlight vaporizer, proceed as for the previous recipes, adjusting the quantity of essential oil accordingly.

Sweet dreams

1 Neroli 2, lavender 2, clary sage 1.

2 Chamomile 2, rose 4.

3 Frankincense 3, mandarin 3.

Meditation

1 Frankincense 3, cedarwood 2, sandalwood 1.

2 Cedarwood 4, cypress 2.

3 Frankincense 3, galbanum 2, elemi 1.

Tranquillity

1 Vetiver 2, clary sage 2, lavender 2.

2 Juniper 3, bergamot 2, cedarwood 2.

3 Galbanum 2, lavender 4.

Blithe spirit (happiness)

1 Geranium 2, palmarosa 3.

2 Rose 3, lemon 1, bergamot 2.

3 Lime 2, graperfruit 2, ylang ylang 2.

Clear mind (for study purposes)

1 Basil 2, rosemary 4.

2 Pine 4, rosemary 2.

3 Peppermint 2, eucalyptus 2, lemon 2.

Passion

1 Ylang ylang 2, rose 3.

2 Patchouli 2, clary sage 2, angelica 2.

3 Carnation 1, sandalwood 2, coriander 3.

Aromatic decoctions

A decoction is an aqueous extraction of hard or woody plant material. Although usually taken as a herbal medicine (just like herb tea), I have discovered that aromatic decoctions can also be used in the nightlight vaporizer to perfume rooms. Choose highly aromatic plant material such as whole cloves, dried ginger root, a cinnamon stick, cardamom seeds or a vanilla pod. If strong enough, a spicy decoction can be vaporized just as it is, or it can be made more aromatic and interesting by adding a few drops of essential oil. As a variation, most spicy decoctions smell wonderful blended 50/50 with orange flower water or rosewater. Moreover, if the spices suit your needs, they can also be used as a base for dosha balancing blends.

You will need approximately 2 rounded teaspoons of dried plant material (e.g. coriander seed, juniper berries, whole cloves) to 240 ml water.

Caution: the aromatic decoctions suggested here are twice as strong as those advocated for internal dosage, so it is not advisable to administer these as medicine.

If possible, roughly grind the spices (except cloves) in a coffee grinder or food processor for a couple of seconds to help release their volatile oils. Put the plant material and water into a small stainless steel, enamel or Pyrex saucepan with a tightly fitting lid. Bring to the boil and simmer *for no more than five minutes*, otherwise the mixture will boil away. Turn off the heat, leave tightly covered and allow to stand overnight. Next day, pour the decoction through some muslin or a fine mesh tea strainer, then funnel into a glass bottle, seal and *store in the fridge, but use within one or two months.*

Other plant material needs to be prepared thus:

Ginger – bruise a dried root by hitting with a wooden mallet or the end of a rolling pin before proceeding as above.

Cinnamon stick – a quarter of a stick will be enough for 240 ml water.

Nutmeg – grate a quarter of a whole nutmeg into 240 ml water.

Vanilla pod – cut one vanilla pod into small pieces, then proceed as above. Alternatively, you could use natural vanilla essence (available from a health shop or delicatessen). Add ½–1 teaspoon to every 50 ml water.

Suggested blends

1 50 ml clove decoction, 50 ml rosewater.

2 25 ml clove decoction, 25 ml cinnamon decoction, 50 ml orange flower water.

3 100 ml vanilla decoction (or 2 teaspoons vanilla extract to 100 ml water), 6 drops ylang ylang, 4 drops lime.

4 50 ml vanilla decoction (or 2 teaspoons vanilla extract in 100 ml water), 25 ml rosewater, 25 ml clove decoction.

5 50 ml cardamom (or nutmeg) decoction, 50 ml orange flower water, 4 drops petitgrain, 4 drops orange.

6 50 ml ginger decoction, 50 ml orange flower water, 8 drops patchouli.

7 25 ml ginger decoction, 75 ml clove (or nutmeg) decoction, 10 drops grapefruit.

8 50 ml coriander decoction, 50 ml juniper decoction, 10 drops bergamot.

9 100 ml cinnamon decoction, 4 drops rose, 4 drops sandalwood.

10 50 ml cinnamon decoction, 50 ml clove decoction, 2 drops ylang ylang, 2 drops neroli, 6 drops mandarin.

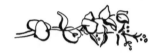

A fragrant harvest of festivals

With the hurly burly pace of modern life, whose heart beats within the metropolis rather than the depths of the rural landscape, we barely have time to 'sit and stare', much less to celebrate the cycle of life, death and rebirth as reflected in the changing seasons. In earlier times, the major seasonal festivals were always celebrated around the time of the spring and autumn equinoxes (when day and night are of equal length) and around the shortest and longest days of the midwinter and midsummer solstices. All these sacred festivals have now been assimilated into Christianity; the midsummer festival has become St John's day; the spring festival as Easter (a movable festival, falling on the first Sunday after the full moon which happens upon or following the spring equinox); Michaelmas and Harvest Festival are around the autumn equinox; and the midwinter celebration has become Christmas.

Whether you choose to celebrate the seasons (or the traditional holy days) with a party, a family get-together, a long walk in the countryside — perhaps to visit an ancient site — or simply with quiet reverence, vaporizing the appropriate aromas in your home can evoke a sense of the sacred. Of course, you may simply wish to vaporize aromatic oils for the sheer joy of breathing in the scents of nature, but whatever the focus, pleasant aromas can certainly enhance the atmosphere of any celebration.

The following room scents will serve as a starting point from which you may develop your own ideas. The first recipe within each group is a water-based blend, i.e. around 20 drops of essential oil to every 100–125 ml water. The second recipe in each section is a simple undiluted essential oil mixture which can be added directly to the water-filled reservoir of the nightlight vaporizer, the molten wax of a candle or the ceramic plate or filter of the electric vaporizer.

Spring Equinox

The beginning of the light half of the year, falling on 21st March in the northern hemisphere and 23rd September in the southern hemisphere. Otherwise, celebrate this festival at Easter. Choose fresh fragrances which suggest spring flowers and awakening woodlands: clary sage, geranium, juniper, lavender, mimosa, palmarosa, petitgrain, pine, rosemary. For an Easter celebration, you could also include the traditional flavours/aromas of vanilla and cinnamon.

1 *Water-based blend* – geranium 3, lavender 6, juniper 4, clary sage 6.

2 *Neat essential oil blend* – mimosa 3, lavender 2, palmarosa 1.

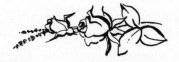

Beltane (May Day)

This is the great Celtic festival of the beginning of summer which is celebrated on May Eve. Beltane is traditionally a festival of youth and love. When the hilltop bonfires had died down, late in the night couples would wander off to the greenwood and make love as the sun rose, a symbolic act of self-empowerment, ensuring the fertility of the land. Choose sensuous oils of intoxicating flowers combined with those suggestive of the greenwood: carnation, cedarwood, clary sage, galbanum, jasmine, neroli, oakmoss, orange flower absolute, rose, sandalwood, vetiver, ylang ylang.

1 *Water-based blend* – jasmine 5, oakmoss 3, clary sage 5, sandalwood 5.

2 *Neat essential oil blend* – rose 3, cedarwood 2, ylang ylang 1.

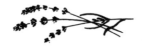

Summer Solstice

The Midsummer festivities traditionally begin around sunset on 20th June in the northern hemisphere and 21st December in the southern hemisphere, with the following sunrise marking the solstice. It is the time of the longest day and shortest night. The most appropriate essences to vaporize at midsummer are those which astrologers have traditionally assigned to the sun. These include angelica, bergamot, black pepper, chamomile, cinnamon, clove, ginger, juniper, lemon, orange and rosemary.

1 *Water-based blend* – angelica 3, bergamot 9, clove 2, orange 5.

2 *Neat essential oil blend* – juniper 3, bergamot 3.

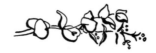

Autumn Equinox

The time of the harvest festival and the beginning of the dark half of the year, falling on, or a few days after, the 21st of September in the northern hemisphere and 21st March in the southern (refer to the current calendar). Sometimes this festival is celebrated at Harvest Moon, when the full moon of the autumn equinox hangs low and huge in the sky, and whose light enables the harvest to continue well after sunset. Choose oils which are evocative of the bountiful earth and of luscious fruits: angelica, bergamot, cardamom, cedarwood, coriander, frankincense, galbanum, grapefruit, lemon, lime, mandarin, orange, patchouli, sandalwood, vetiver.

1 *Water-based blend* – frankincense 6, angelica 2, mandarin 5, bergamot 5.

2 *Neat essential oil blend* – coriander 2, bergamot 2, patchouli 2.

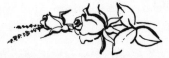

Samhain or Hallowe'en

The feast of the summer's end and the Celtic New Year's Eve, traditionally celebrated after dusk on 31st October. In the Christian calendar it is All Saints' Day, falling on 1st November. Samhain (pronounced sa-in) is also a festival of remembrance for the dead, and the night when the veil between our world and the Otherworld is thinnest, thus communication with the Great Ones becomes possible. Choose dark and mysterious essences such as galbanum, patchouli or vetiver, heightened with evergreen oils such as cedarwood, cypress, juniper, oakmoss and pine. To bridge the 'two worlds', add a touch of clary sage.

1 *Water-based blend* – vetiver 3, juniper 5, cedarwood 5, clary sage 6.

2 *Neat essential oil blend* – oakmoss 2, galbanum 1, clary sage 3.

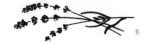

Winter Solstice

The time of the shortest day and the longest night when the sun is at its southernmost point in the sky in the northern hemisphere, on the eve of the 21st of December. Of course, the midwinter festival in the northern hemisphere is also celebrated as Christmas. In the southern hemisphere the Winter Solstice falls on 21st June. Choose rich, warming essences of resins, spices and citrus: bergamot, cardamom, cinnamon, clove, coriander, elemi, frankincense, ginger, juniper, mandarin, myrrh, orange. You may also wish to include pine in your midwinter blends, which harmonizes well with resins or with citrus.

1 *Water-based blend* – cardamom 3, clove 3, mandarin 6, bergamot 6.

2 *Neat essential oil blend* – frankincense 3, cinnamon 1, orange 2.

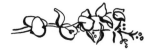

Other celebrations

Whatever the occasion, be it a wedding anniversary, a candlelit dinner à deux, a child's birthday party, or perhaps a house-warming party, nature's essential oils can always be summoned to work their special magic, thus creating an ambience of enchantment.

And remember, you really don't need a special occasion as an excuse to enjoy and benefit from the therapeutic powers of essential oils – make them part of your everyday life.

Bibliography

Ackerman, D. *A Natural History of the Senses*,
Chapmans, 1990

Chopra, D. *Perfect Health*, Bantam Books, 1990

Chopra D. *Quantum Healing*, Bantam Books, 1989

Fischer-Rizzi, S. *Complete Aromatherapy Handbook*,
Sterling, 1990

Gattefosse, R. *Formulary of Perfumes and Cosmetics*,
Chemical Publishing, 1959

Jellinek, Dr P. *The Practice of Modern Perfumery*,
Leonard Hill, 1959

Kennett, F. *The History of Perfume*, Harrap, 1975

Lake, M. *Scents and Sensuality*, Futura, 1989

Lawless, J. *The Encyclopaedia of Essential Oils*,
Element Books, 1992

Maple, E. *The Magic of Perfume*, Aquarian Press, 1973

Ryman, D. *Aromatherapy – The Encyclopedia of Plants
and Oils*, Piatkus, 1990

Slade, P. *Natural Magic, A Seasonal Guide*, Hamlyn, 1990

Tisserand, R. *Aromatherapy for Everyone*, Penguin, 1990

Tucker Fettner, A. *Potpourri*, Hutchinson, 1977

Van Toller, S. and Dodds G. *Perfumery, The Psychology
and Biology of Fragrance*, Chapman and Hall, 1988

Watts, M. *Plant Aromatics* (privately published),
Whitham, 1992

Wildwood, C. *Aromatherapy and Massage*,
Element Books 1992

Wildwood, C. *Creative Aromatherapy*, Thorsons, 1993

Wildwood, C. *Holistic Aromatherapy*, Thorsons, 1992

Worwood, V.A. *Fragrant Pharmacy*, Bantam Press 1990

Useful Addresses

The following mail order suppliers stock a range of high quality essential oils and vaporizing equipment.

UK
Kittywake Oils
Cae Kitty, Taliaris, Llandeilo, Dyfed SA19 7DP
Butterbur and Sage
101 Highgrove Street, Reading, Berkshire RG1 5EJ
Purple Flame Aromatics
61 Clinton Lane, Kenilworth, Warwickshire CV8 1AS
Aqua Oleum
Unit 3, Lower Wharf, Wall Bridge, Stroud
Gloucestershire GL5 3JA
Fleur Aromatherapy
Pembroke Studios, Pembroke Road, London NIO 2JE
Verde
45 Northcote Road, London SW11 6PJ

USA
Aroma Vera Inc
PO Box 3609, Culver City, California 90231
M Das Co
888 Brannan Street, San Francisco, CA 94103

Australia
Margaret Tozer – Australian School of Awareness
251 Dorset Road, Croydon, Victoria 3136

South Africa
Lucile Bischoff
PO Box 743, Gallo Manor, 2052

Index

Principal references are given in **bold type.**

absolute oils, 20–1
Ackerman, Diane, 7
aftershave, 100–1
ajowan, xiv
alcohol as carrier, 59, 61, 87
  for floral waters, 98
allergy to perfume, xiii
almond, bitter, xiv
almond oil, xiii, 24, 62
amber, xvi
ambergris, xvi, 72
ambrette, 73
Amoore, J.E., 5
amyris (West Indian sandalwood), 52
Ancient Egyptian perfumes, 12–13
androsterone secretion, 74
angelica, **26–7**, 81
  perfume note, 69
animal oils, 72, 85
aniseed, xiv
anosmia, 6–7
aphrodisiac blends, 72–5
  love potions, 94–5
applying perfume, 96–7
aromatic waters *see* floral waters/colognes
asarone, 12

atlas cedarwood *see* cedarwood
atomizers, 99
autumn equinox, 125
Avicenna, 13
avocado oil, 62
Ayurvedic approach, 107–15

balsam of Peru, xiv
basil, **27**
  with bergamot, 27, 28
  perfume note, 69
  as room scent, 81
  toxicity/skin reactions, xvi
bath oils, 80
beard perfumes, 88
beeswax, 60, 61
  in solid perfumes, 95–6
Beltane (May Day), 123–4
benzoin, 71
bergamot, **28**
  with basil, 27, 28
  with cedarwood, 30
  with chamomile, 31
  with clary sage, 28, 32
  with cypress, 28, 34
  effect on mood, 71

with geranium, 28, 38
with juniper, 40
with marjoram, 43
with patchouli, 47, 56
perfume note, 66, 67, 68, 69
with petitgrain, 49
with pine, 49
with sandalwood, 52
shelf life, 24
therapeutic uses, 18, 28
birch, toxicity of, xiv
Birnberg, Judith R., 7
black pepper, **28–9**, 81
cns effect, 18
effect on mood, 72
perfume note, 69
with sandalwood, 29, 52
body scents (pheromones), 8–9
Bois de Rose, 23
boldo leaf, xiv
Bonaparte, Napoleon I, 14, 73
bottles for storage, 24, 25, 63
breastfeeding, xiv
broom (Spanish), xv
buchu, xv

cabbage rose *see* rose
cajeput, 18
calamus, xv
camphor, 71
stereochemical theory, 6

toxicity of, xv
candles (scented), 105–6
cannabis resin scent, 71
caraway, 15
carbon dioxide extraction, 21
cardamom, **29**, 81
decoctions, 121
with grapefruit, 39
perfume note, 69
as room scent, 62
carnation, **29–30**, 82
with cedarwood, 30
effect on mood, 71
mock concentrate, 91, 93–4
perfume note, 67, 68, 70
purchasing, 26
cassia, xvii
cedarwood, **30**
with cardamom, 29
with carnation, 30
concentrates, 91–2
as embalming aromatic, 12
with eucalyptus, 35
with frankincense, 30, 36
with ginger, 38
historical aspects, 75
with marjoram, 43
with palmarosa, 47
with patchouli, 47
perfume note, 70
with pine, 49
storage of, 24
celebrations/festivals, 122–6

chamomile, **31**, 81
  essence consistency, 15
  with marjoram, 43
  as massage oil, 79
  with neroli, 31, 45
  perfume note, 69
  therapeutic properties,
    17, 18
Chanel, Gabrielle (Coco),
  14–15
Chanel No 5, x, 14–15
chervil, xv
Chopra, Deepak, 107
Christmas time, 126
chrysanthemum, 2
chypre scents, 85
  from the wildwood, 89
cinnamon, **31–2**, 59, 81
  with cardamom, 29
  decoctions, 122
  effect on mood, 72
  with elemi, 35
  with frankincense, 31, 36
  irritant to skin, xv
  perfume note, 69
  as room scent, 62
citronella, 17
citrus oils, 17
  with angelica, 27
  with black pepper, 29
  with cardamom, 29
  with carnation, 30
  with cinnamon, 31
  citrus concentrates, 93
  with clove, 33
  with coriander, 33

  with cypress, 34
  with elemi, 35
  with frankincense, 36
  with geranium, 38
  with ginger, 38
  with grapefruit, 39
  with jasmine, 39
  with juniper, 40
  with lemon, 41
  with lime, 42
  with mandarin, 42
  with myrrh, 44
  with neroli, 45
  with orange, 46
  with rose otto, 50
  shelf life, 24
  see also under specific oils
clary sage, xvii, **32**, 56
  with angelica, 27
  with basil, 27
  with bergamot, 28, 32
  with carnation, 30
  with cedarwood, 30
  with chamomile, 31
  with cypress, 34
  with geranium, 32, 38
  with jasmine, 32, 39
  with lime, 42
  with neroli, 45
  with oakmoss, 32, 46
  with orange, 46
  with patchouli, 47
  perfume note, 66, 67, 69
  with petitgrain, 49
  synesthesia and, 6
  therapeutic uses, 17, 32

with vetiver, 53
clove, **32–3**, 59
  with cardamom, 29
  effect on mood, 72
  with elemi, 35
  with geranium, 38
  irritant to skin, xv
  with patchouli, 47
  perfume note, 69
  with petitgrain, 49
  phenols in, 18
  as room scent, 62, 69, 81
  with sandalwood, 52
  with vanilla, 33, 52
coconut oil, 60–1, 62, 86
Coleridge, Samuel, 2
colognes *see* floral
    waters/colognes
colours and fragrances, 3, 6
  colour-rosette test, 76–8
concentrates, 91–4
conditioning (odour), 10
coriander, **33**
  with bergamot, 28
  with carnation, 30
  with clary sage, 32
  decoctions, 122
  effect on mood, 72
  with elemi, 35
  with ginger, 38
  with grapefruit, 39
  with mimosa, 44
  with neroli, 45
  perfume note, 69
  as room scent, 62
cost/purchasing 26, 55

costus root, 73
coumarin, 14
cumin, xv
cypress, **34**
  with bergamot, 28, 34
  with cedarwood, 30
  with coriander, 33
  with eucalyptus, 35
  with grapefruit, 39
  with juniper, 34, 40
  with marjoram, 34, 43
  with myrrh, 44
  perfume note, 70
  sad fragrance, 2

de-ionized water, 61, 87
decoctions, 120–2
deertongue, xv
Dioscorides, 12
distillation process, 19–23
  history of, 13
  home distillation, 21–3
distilled water, 61, 87
Dodd, George, 7
Dreams of Mandalay
    perfume, 90

eau de cologne *see* floral
    waters/colognes
Egyptian perfumes, 12–13
elecampane, xv
electric fragrancer, 63,
    103–4
elemi, **34–5**, 81

with bergamot, 28
with juniper, 40
perfume note, 70
embalming in Ancient
    Egypt, 12
endorphins, 4
enfleurage, 20
enkephalins, 4
erogenic/aphrodisiac oils,
    71, 72–5
love potions, 94–5
eucalyptus, 15, **35**, 81
    effect on mood, 71, 72
    with lemon, 35, 41
    with marjoram, 35, 43
    with peppermint, 48
    perfume note, 69
    with pine, 35, 49
    therapeutic properties,
        18, 35
European perfumes, 13–15
extraction processes, 19–23

facial oils, 79, 80
fennel, **35–6**, 81
    perfume note, 69
    with sandalwood, 36, 52
    therapeutic uses, 17, 35
festivals/holidays, 122–6
floral scents, 85
    Flowers of Eden, 89
    stereochemical theory,
        5–6
floral waters/colognes, 19,
    61, 85, **97–9**

lavender water, 19, 61
orange flower water, 45,
    61, 97, 100
perfume notes, 68
shelf lives, 25
see also rosewater
Flowers of Eden perfume, 89
foods:
    Ayurveda principles and,
        109–11
    body scent and, 8–9
Fougère Royale, 14
Four Thieves' Vinegar, 14
fragrancer (electric), 63,
    103–4
Frangipani, 13
frankincense, **36**, 81
    with basil, 27
    with bergamot, 28
    with cardamom, 29
    with carnation, 30
    with cedarwood, 30, 36
    chemical content, 16
    with cinnamon, 31, 36
    with clary sage, 32
    with coriander, 33
    effect on mood, 71
    with elemi, 35
    with ginger, 38
    historical aspects, 11, 12,
        75
    with lemon, 41
    as massage oil, 79
    with myrrh, 44
    with orange, 46
    perfume note, 70

psychoactive properties, 11
vintage, 24, 36
French basil *see* basil
From the wildwood perfume, 89

galbanum, **37**, 81
  with juniper, 40
  perfume note, 69
garlic, synesthesia and, 6
gas chromatography, 16–17
geranium, **37–8**, 82
  with basil, 27
  with bergamot, 28, 38
  with chamomile, 31
  with clary sage, 32, 38
  with fennel, 36
  with galbanum, 37
  with grapefruit, 39
  with juniper, 38, 40
  with myrrh, 44
  with palmarosa, 47
  with patchouli, 38, 47, 56
  perfume note, 67, 69
  with petitgrain, 49
  therapeutic uses, 18, 37
gifts of perfumes, 101
ginger, **38**, 81
  with bergamot, 28
  with carnation, 30
  decoctions, 120–1
  effect on mood, 72
  perfume note, 69

grapefruit, **38–9**
  perfume note, 69
grapeseed oil, xiii, 62
Grasse, 13–14
Great Plague, 14
green scents, 85
    green concentrates, 92
    Of the glade perfume, 90

hair perfume, 87–8
Hallowe'en, 125–6
hallucinogens:
  asarone, 12
  synesthesia and, 3
happiness chemicals, 4, 5
holidays/festivals, 122–6
hyacinth, 71
hyssop, xv, 18

inula, xv

jaborandi, xv
jasmine, **39**, 81
  with black pepper, 29
  with cedarwood, 30
  with chamomile, 31
  with clary sage, 32, 39
  with coriander, 33
  effect on mood, 71
  enfleurage extraction, 20
  with geranium, 38
  in modern perfumery, 15
  with neroli, 45

organic, 23
perfume note, 67, 68, 70
with petitgrain, 49
with sandalwood, 39, 52
therapeutic uses, 17, 39
with vetiver, 53
vintage, 24
Je Reviens perfume, 14
jojoba oil, 60, 61, 86
juniper, 40
   with cedarwood, 30
   with clary sage, 32
   with coriander, 33
   with cypress, 34, 40
   with geranium, 38, 40
   with lemon, 41
   with myrrh, 44
   perfume note, 69, 70
   with pine, 40, 49

Kipling, Rudyard, 2
Kyphi (Egyptian incense),
   12

lavender, 40–1
   as antiseptic, 16, 17–18
   with bergamot, 28
   with black pepper, 29
   with chamomile, 31
   with clary sage, 32
   with cypress, 34
   effect on mood, 71
   with elemi, 35
   essence consistency, 15
   with eucalyptus, 35
   with fennel, 36
   with galbanum, 37
   with geranium, 38
   with grapefruit, 39
   with juniper, 40
   with lime, 42
   with marjoram, 43
   as massage oil, 79
   with mimosa, 44
   with myrrh, 44
   with neroli, 45
   with oakmoss, 46
   oil sites in plant, 15–16
   oil yields, 16
   with orange, 46
   with patchouli, 47, 56
   with peppermint, 48
   perfume note, 67, 68, 69,
      70
   with petitgrain, 49
   with pine, 49
   with sandalwood, 52
   therapeutic uses, 16, 17,
      18, 40
   with vetiver, 53, 56
lavender water, 19, 61
lemon, 41
   with chamomile, 31
   effect on mood, 71
   with eucalyptus, 35, 41
   with peppermint, 48
   perfume note, 66
   with pine, 49
   therapeutic uses, 17, 18,
      42

lemongrass, 17, 81
  effect on mood, 71
  perfume note, 69
light bulb perfumery,
    104—5
limbic system, 4
lime, **41—2**, 82
  with basil, 27
  effect on mood, 71
  perfume note, 69
  with vanilla, 52
loss of smell (anosmia), 6—7
love potions, 94—5
LSD (hallucinogen), 3

mail order suppliers, 23—4,
    128
mandarin, **42—3**
  perfume note, 69
marjoram, **43**
  with cypress, 34, 43
  with eucalyptus, 35, 43
  with peppermint, 48
  perfume note, 70
  with pine, 49
  therapeutic uses, 17, 43
massage oils, 62, **79—80**
  storage time, 25
Medici, Catherine de, 13
melissa oil, xvi
metric conversions, 64—5
midsummer festivals, 124
mimosa, **43—4**, 82
  perfume note, 70
  purchasing, 26

sad fragrance, 2
  with sandalwood, 44, 52
  with vetiver, 53
minty odours,
    stereochemical theory,
    6
Montaigne, 2
mood-enhancing effects,
    71—2
  aphrodisiacs, 72—5
  love potions, 94—5
  room scents, 116—19
mugwort, xv, 17
music and colours, 3
musk, 14
musk seed, 73
myrrh, **44**, 81
  chemical content, 16
  with elemi, 35
  for embalming, 12
  essence consistency, 15
  with neroli, 45
  with orange, 46
  perfume note, 70

names of perfumes, 101—2
Napoleon I, 14, 73
narcissus, xv, 71, 73
Natural History of the Senses
    (Ackerman), 6—7
neroli, **44—5**, 81
  with basil, 27
  with bergamot, 28
  with cedarwood, 30
  with chamomile, 31, 45

dilution of, 24
effect on mood, 71
erogenic component, 71
with geranium, 38
with ginger, 38
with grapefruit, 39
with lime, 42
with mandarin, 42
as massage oil, 79
with mimosa, 44
with oakmoss, 46
with orange, 46
with patchouli, 47
perfume note, 67, 69, 70
with petitgrain, 49
purchasing, 26
tampering of, 23
with vanilla, 52
nutmeg, 18
decoctions, 121

oakmoss, **45–6**, 82
with angelica, 27
with basil, 27
with chamomile, 31
with clary sage, 32, 46
with galbanum, 37
with juniper, 40
with lemon, 41
with mimosa, 44
mock concentrate, 91, 92
with myrrh, 44
with palmarosa, 47
with patchouli, 47
perfume note, 66, 68, 70
with petitgrain, 46, 49

with sandalwood, 52
with vetiver, 53
vintage, 24, 45
Of the glade perfume, 90
oil burner, 63, 103, 106, 107
olfactory sense mechanisms, 3–4
olive oil, synesthesia and, 6
opiates, natural, 4–5
Opium (perfume), x
opium smoke, scent of, 71
orange, **46**
enfleurage extraction, 20
perfume note, 69
orange flower absolute, 45, 81
effect on mood, 71
perfume note, 70
with petitgrain, 49
orange flower water, 19, 45, 61, 97
as aftershave base, 100
oregano, xv, 18
organically produced essences, 23
oriental scents, 85–6
Dreams of Mandalay perfume, 90

palmarosa, **47**
chemical content, 18
with grapefruit, 39
perfume note, 69, 70
with petitgrain, 49

Parfum Idéal, 14
Parquet, Paul, 14
patch test, xiii
patchouli, **47**, 56, 82
   with angelica, 27
   with geranium, 38, 47
   with ginger, 38
   with myrrh, 44
   perfume note, 66, 68, 70
   with sandalwood, 47, 52
   synesthesia and, 6
   with vetiver, 53
   vintage, 24, 47
pennyroyal, xv, 17
pepper _see_ black pepper
peppermint, **48**, 81
   effect on mood, 72
   perfume note, 69
Perfect Health (D Chopra),
     107
perfumes:
   carriers, 59–61
   derivation of term
     perfume, 11
   equipment, 62–5
   formulae for, 88–101
   as gifts, 101
   ingredients, 61–2
   names of, 101–2
   perfume notes, 66–70, 86
   solid, 61, 95–6
   starter selection, 58–9
Perkin, William Henry, 14
personality and fragrance,
     76–8
petitgrain, **48**–9

   with coriander, 33
   with oakmoss, 46, 49
   perfume note, 69
pheromones, 8–9
Piesse (French perfumier),
     66
pine, **49**
   with clary sage, 32
   with coriander, 33
   with cypress, 34
   effect on mood, 71
   with eucalyptus, 35, 49
   with galbanum, 37
   with juniper, 40, 49
   with myrrh, 44
   perfume note, 69, 70
   therapeutic properties, 17
plague, 14
plastic bottles/jars, 63
pregnancy, xiv
price aspects, x, 55
Proust, Marcel, 2
psycho-active substances:
   in frankincense, 11
   synesthesia and, 3
   Theriaque, 12
psycho-aromatherapy chart,
     116–19
pulse points, 96

resin concentrates, 93
resinoid oils, 20–1
Rimski-Korsakov, 3
Roman chamomile _see_
    chamomile

room scents, 57, 58, 82,
    103–26
  as gifts, 101
rose, 15, **49–50**, 81
  aphrodisiac component,
      71, 73
  with black pepper, 29
  with cedarwood, 30
  with chamomile, 31
  with clove, 33
  effect on mood, 71
  with ginger, 38
  with mimosa, 44
  in modern perfumery, 15
  with neroli, 45
  with oakmoss, 46
  organic, 23
  with patchouli, 47
  perfume note, 66, 68, 69,
      70
  with sandalwood, 50, 52
  synesthesia and, 6
  synthetic counterpart, x
  therapeutic properties, 17
  with vanilla, 52
  with vetiver, 53
rose otto, 50, 81
  consistency, 15
  as massage oil, 79
  perfume note, 67, 68, 69,
      70
  purchasing, 26
  rosewater, 19, 50, 61
  therapeutic uses, 18, 50
  vintage, 24, 50
rosemary, 15, **50–1**

  with black pepper, 29
  with cedarwood, 30, 51
  effect on mood, 71, 72
  with elemi, 35
  with eucalyptus, 35
  with grapefruit, 39
  with juniper, 40
  with lime, 42
  with marjoram, 43
  with peppermint, 48, 51
  perfume note, 70
  with petitgrain, 49, 51
  with pine, 49, 51
  therapeutic uses, 18, 51
  used by Napoleon, 14,
      73
rosewater, 19, 50, 61, 97
  as aftershave base, 100
  effect on mood, 73
rosewood, 23
rue, xvii

sad fragrances, 2
sage, xv, 17
Samhain festival, 125–6
Sand, George, 2
sandalwood, **51–2**, 57, 82
  anosmia to, 7
  with black pepper, 29, 52
  concentrates, 91–2
  with coriander, 33
  with cypress, 34
  with fennel, 36, 52
  with frankincense, 36
  with geranium, 38

with ginger, 38
historical aspects, 75
with jasmine, 39, 52
with juniper, 40
as massage oil, 79
with mimosa, 44, 52
with myrrh, 44
with palmarosa, 47
with patchouli, 47, 52
perfume note, 66, 68, 70
with rose, 50, 52
with rose otto, 50
with vanilla, 52
versus amyris, 52
with vetiver, 52, 53
vintage, 24, 51
santolina, xvi
sassafras, xvi
savine, xvi
savory, xvi
Schiller, J., 2
Scotch pine *see* pine
Scriabin, Alexander, 3
shelf lives, 24–5, 87
smell-testing, 82–3
smelling strips, 62
smelling technique, 56–8
solid perfumes, 61, 95–6
soya oil, 62
Spanish sage, xv
spice oils:
aromatic decoctions, 97, 120–2
with black pepper, 29
with cinnamon, 31
with clove, 33

with frankincense, 36
with mandarin, 42
with myrrh, 44
with orange, 46
as splash-ons, 97
see also under specific spice
spices (whole), 62
spikenard, 12
spring equinox, 123
steam distillation, 19, 21
stereochemical theory of odour, 5–6
storage aspects, 24–5, 87
stream diffuser, 104
summer solstice, 124
sunflower oil, xiii, 62
suppliers, 23–4, 128–9
sweet fennel *see* fennel
sweet marjoram *see* marjoram
synesthesia, 3, 6
synethetic fragrances, ix–xi

tagetes, 81
perfume note, 69
tansy, xvi, 17
tarrogon, xvi
tea tree, 18
terminal illness, 5
therapeutic properties of oils, 17–19
aromatic baths, 80
see also specific oils
Theriaque, 12
thuja, xvi

thyme, 18
tonka bean, xvi, 73
toxic oils, xiv–xvi
tuberose, 20, 71, 73

valerian, 73, 83
Valnet, Jean, 13
Van Toller, Steve, 7
vanilla, **52**
  with clove, 33, 52
  decoctions, 121
  effect on mood, 18, 71
  home-made oil, 91, 94
  perfume note, 70
  vanilla pod, 62
vaporizer (oil burner), 63,
    103, 106, 107
vetiver, 15, **53**, 56, 82
  with angelica, 27
  with cedarwood, 30
  with clary sage, 32, 53
  with frankincense, 36
  with ginger, 38
  with patchouli, 47, 53
  perfume note, 66, 67, 70
  with sandalwood, 52, 53
  with vanilla, 52
violet, 2, 71

water (distilled), 61, 87
West Indian sandalwood,
    52
winter solstice, 126
wintergreen, xvi
wormseed, xvi
wormwood, xvi, 17
writers, influence of scent
    on, 2

ylang ylang, **53–4**, 82
  with cedarwood, 30
  with chamomile, 31
  with clove, 33
  effect on mood, 71
  with galbanum, 37
  with lime, 42
  with mimosa, 44
  with neroli, 45
  organic production, 23
  perfume note, 67, 68, 70
  with vanilla, 52
  with vetiver, 53, 54
Youth Dew, x

PIATKUS BOOKS

If you have enjoyed reading this book, you may be interested in other titles published by Piatkus. These include:

Health and Healing

Acupressure: How to Cure Common Ailments the Natural Way Michael Reed Gach

The Alexander Technique Liz Hodgkinson

Aromatherapy: The Encyclopedia of Plants and Oils and How They Help You Daniele Ryman

Art as Medicine: Creating a Therapy of the Imagination Shaun McNiff

Arthritis Relief at Your Fingertips: How to Use Acupressure Massage to Ease Your Aches and Pains Michael Reed Gach

Be Your Own Best Friend: How to Achieve Greater Self-Esteem and Happiness Louis Proto

The Encyclopedia of Alternative Health Care Kristin Olsen

The Good Health Food Guide: Which Foods and Supplements Will Boost Your Health Dr Eric Trimmer

Healing Breakthroughs: How Your Attitudes and Beliefs Can Affect Your Health Dr Larry Dossey

Herbal Remedies: The Complete Guide to Natural Healing Jill Nice

Homeopathic Medicine for Children and Infants Dana Ullman

Increase Your Energy Louis Proto

Iridology: How to Discover Your Own Pattern of Health and Well-Being Through the Eye Dorothy Hall

Look Younger, Feel Better Dr James Scala and Barbara Jacques

Mind Power: Use Positive Thinking to Change Your life Christian H. Godefroy

Off the Hook: How to Break Free from Addiction and Enjoy a New Way of Life Corinne Sweet

The Reflexology Handbook Laura Norman and Thomas Cowan

Self-Healing: Use Your Mind to Heal Your Body Louis Proto

The Shiatsu Workbook: A Beginner's Guide Nigel Dawes

Spiritual Healing Liz Hodgkinson

Stress Control Through Self-Hypnosis Dr Arthur Jackson

Super Health: How to Activate and Control Your Body's Natural Defences Christian H. Godefroy

Super Massage Gordon Inkeles

Teach Yourself to Meditate Eric Harrison

The Three Minute Meditator David Harp with Nina Feldman

Women's Cancers: The Treatment Options Donna Dawson

Working With Your Chakras Ruth White

Your Healing Power: A Comprehensive Guide to Channelling Your Healing Energies Jack Angelo

Mind, Body and Spirit

Ambika's Guide to Healing and Wholeness: The Energetic Guide to the Chakras and Colour Ambika Wauters

As I See It: A Psychic's Guide to Developing Your Sensing and Healing Abilities Betty F. Balcombe

Awakening to Change: Your Guide to Personal Empowerment in the New Millennium Soozi Holbeche

Care of the Soul: How to Add Depth and Meaning to Everyday Life Thomas Moore

Chinese Elemental Astrology E A Crawford and Teresa Kennedy

Colour Your Life: Discover Your True Personality Through Colour Howard and Dorothy Sun

Creating Abundance: How to Bring Wealth and Fulfilment into Your Life Andrew Ferguson

The Energy Connection: Simple Answers to Life's Important Questions Betty F Balcombe

The I Ching or Book of Changes: A Guide to Life's Turning Points Brian Browne Walker

Inward Bound: Exploring the Geography of Your Emotions Sam Keen

Living Magically: A New Vision of Reality Gill Edwards

The Personal Growth Handbook: A Guide to Groups, Movements and Healing Treatments Liz Hodgkinson

A Pocketful of Dreams Denise Linn

The Power of Gems and Crystals Soozi Holbeche

The Power of Your Dreams Soozi Holbeche

Rituals for Everyday Living: Special Ways to Mark Important Events in Your Life Lorna St Aubyn

The Secret World of Your Dreams Julia and Derek Parker

Spiritual Healing Liz Hodgkinson

Stepping into the Magic: A New Approach to Everyday Living Gill Edwards

Transform Your Life: A Step-by-Step Programme Diana Cooper

For a free brochure with further information on our full range of titles, please write to:

Piatkus Books
Freepost 7 (WD 4505)
London W1E 4EZ

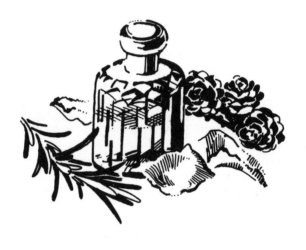